Common Problems of Children

Published by :
Lotus Press Publishers & Distributors

Common Problems of Children

[A Handbook for all Parents and Teachers to Tackle Contemporary Problems Relating to Children]

Chitra Garg
M.A., B.Ed.

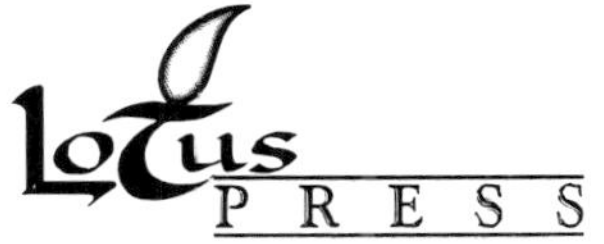

4735/22, Prakash Deep Building
Ansari Road, Darya Ganj,
New Delhi - 110002

Lotus Press : Publishers & Distributors
Unit No. 220, 2nd Floor, 4735/22, Prakash Deep Building,
Ansari Road, Darya Ganj, New Delhi- 110002
Ph.: 23280047, 98118-38000
• E-mail : lotuspress1984@gmail.com
www.lotuspress.co.in

Common Problems of Children

ISBN : 81-8382-156-1 (PB)

Printed & Published by : **Lotus Press Publishers & Distributors,** New Delhi-02

TO THE READERS

Friends

Every young girl and boy dreams of golden future. After marriage every couple dreams of active and smart children in their house. Children are the future citizens of the country. They change the lives of their parents with their love and innocence. But to make them good citizens is the duty of their parents. If they are given right directions, they become disciplined, humble and loving persons.

Sometimes children become obstinate, selfish or rude due to undue love and pamperedness. Many such problems are faced by parents and teachers and it becomes difficult to change the behaviour of such children.

This book has been written to guide parents and teachers who are facing such problems with children. Problems of children may be psychological or behavioural. Mrs. Neena Puri, former Speech and Child Specialist of Children Guidance Centre, Lajpat Nagar IV, (A Government of India Enterprises) has helped me a lot to guide me and write such a book. I have taken consultations of some other doctors also on some related topics. I do hope that this book will be helpful to all parents and teachers.

CHITRA GARG

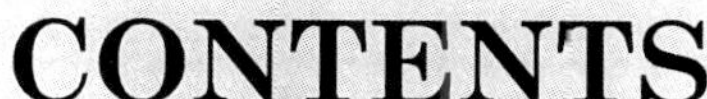

CONTENTS

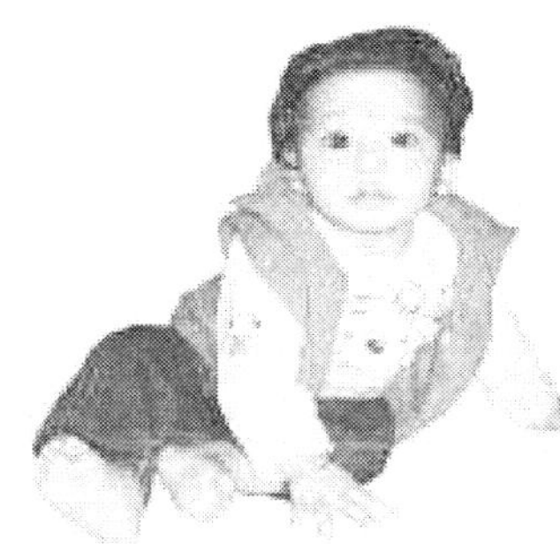

1

A BUNDLE OF JOY: YOUR LITTLE ONE

Parenthood is a cherished dream for one and all. The news of the forthcoming arrival of a young one brings about a drastic and colourful change in the atmosphere of any house. The family members take upon themselves different responsibilities to welcome the new entrant. Grandparents, especially grandmothers get busy in preparing clothes, bedding and other essentials for their new guest–the little one. The excitement doesn't stop here. When the young one arrives, it appears as if spring is in its full bloom. The child becomes the object of attention for each and every member of the family.

A slight whisper or exclamation from the child is enough to capture the attention of the elderly people in the house, (grandparents in most cases) who are ready to attend to him immediately and shower their overwhelming love on the child. The tendency to always shelter or overprotect the child, often takes the form of pampering which in turn manifests in an extreme way in the form of behavioural problems. It so happens that many a times that the family members turn a blind eye towards the misbehaviour of the child because of their overpowering love for him, whereas his misbehaviour is only too apparent before friends, guests and other acquaintances. These guests, by the virtue of their delicate relationship with the parents are unable to express their concerns for the child. They can't discuss the misbehaviour or bad manners of the child before them.

In this time and age, we find parents greatly troubled by the problems associated with their children, but as they are unaware of the root cause of such problems, they are unable to find a solution to them. It is believed that the role of the teachers in the school is similar to the role of the parents perform at home. Therefore, even teachers are confronted with behavioural problems of children on a day-to-day basis; the behavioural problems are in fact, psychological problems, based on child psychology.

Any type of change in the general behaviour of the child is rooted in a pertinent cause. There are some children who are naughty by virtue of their individual nature. Parents should have a thorough knowledge about the need, nature and tendency of their child. This itself will prevent many problems from taking a form. In this book, I have discussed different behavioural problems pertaining to children in detail. I have attempted to focus on the root cause and suggest a solution to these problems as well.

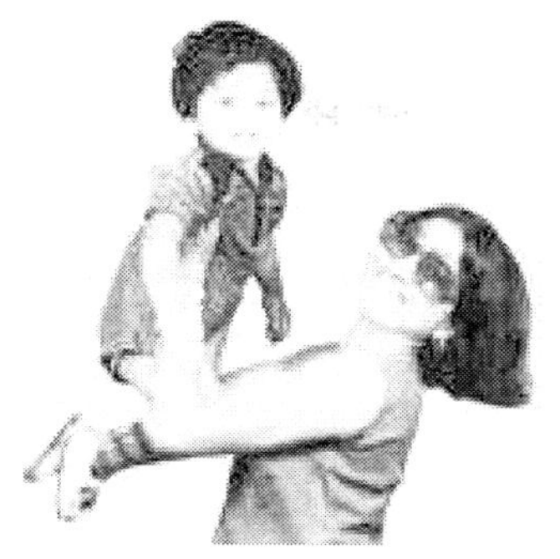

2

WHY EVERY CHILD BEHAVES IN A DIFFERENT WAY?

Child Psychology

Every child completely differs from any another child in terms of his nature and behaviour. Some children are good-natured with a pleasant countenance and never cry, except when they enter into a physical fight with some other child. On the other hand, there are some other children who have a depressed personality, they break into tears at the slightest instance. These children use this very tendency to cry as a means to fulfil their demands. Apart from the above two prototypes, children can be friendly, hardworking, lazy, intelligent, timid, always happy, critic etc.

An infant of three months of age and above starts understanding how he can get his demands fulfilled. However, it would be wrong to conclude the children are selfish and deceiving from this age itself. It is just that the child starts using different ways and means in order to fulfil his requirements. Some parents fulfil each and every necessary and unnecessary demand of the child right from his childhood. This results in the child becoming obstinate and stubborn when he grows up and becomes a major cause for worry for the parents.

CAUSES FOR DIFFERENT REACTIONS AND BEHAVIOUR

- **Difference in inherent nature and upbringing**

The behaviour of the child depends upon his inherent nature to quite some extent. In addition to this, upbringing also prays a very important role on influencing the nature and behaviour of the child. If the parents of the child, specially the mother is timid or faint-hearted and she gets scared at every other thing, such as loud noise, lightning or becomes completely frightened watching horror scenes and starts shivering, hearing the news of accident (mishap), then the child too will be timid when he grows up. If he is successful in overcoming his fears due to the atmosphere in his school or due to any other circumstance, even then the tendency to fear remains subdued in his conscience. It surfaces in the future when such a situation arises.

Child Psychology says that if the children are specifically forbidden to do a certain thing, then they definitely try to do it practically at least once whenever they get an opportunity. For instance, if a 2-3 year old has been told not to put his hand into the mouth of the pet dog as it can bite him, then the child will definitely try it when he is alone with the dog. If the dog happens to bite him, the child will be terrified to go near the dog in the future.

- **The child's desire for first hand experience**

If the child has not been warned that such and such thing is dangerous, he will have no inhibitions in touching it or getting close to it. If you have already not told the child that snakes or certain insects are poisonous, he will fearlessly pick up these things. But the child will immediately understand that going near fire can be dangerous for him. If you forbid the child to touch a hot cup of tea/coffee, he doesn't make an attempt to try it himself. If the child hurts or burns himself or has a bad experience during the first time, he develops a fear for that particular thing forever.

It is fairly normal for small children to put anything to their mouth first. This action symbolises the child's urge to experience the thing. At the time the child is oblivious to fact of whether the thing is edible or not.

The child can easily copy or repeat a work or action he has seen his peer or family member do. However, at the same time if an attempt is made to teach him something separately, he may take a lot of time to learn. If there are two children in a family, then parents have to invest a lot of time in the first child teaching him toilet habits, how to wear his clothes, riding a tricycle and other such things of daily life. But the younger one learns all these things in less time by just observing his sibling do the same.

- **Genetic reasons**

Certain actions or habits are formed in a child out of genetic reasons. Some children are short-tempered, obstinate or very fat from their childhood. It is generally said that girls bear a resemblance to their fathers in looks and behaviour, while boys take after their mothers. Therefore if the child displays extreme anger or any such bad habit, the mother or the grandparents dismiss the habit, attributing genetic reasons for the same. Infact sometimes they feel proud that the child has inherited the family traits.

• Food related habits

The diet and food habits of the child too can be due to his genes. Some children prefer to eat sweets, some like salty snacks, while some love to gorge on very spicy street food. Then people draw comparisons between the food habits of the child with his parents. The reality of the matter is that during his initial days the child is fed things that are liked or eaten by the family. As he grows up and is capable of making his own choices, he chooses his liking from among the different varieties offered to him.

• Health of the child

The health of the child is as important as his habits and food. Children can become plump and overweight if they eat in excess, have very less physical activity, are a couch potato (watch too much T.V.), or if they consume a lot of fast food or sweets etc. Some children are plump from infancy. If the mother or any other close relative is overweight, then it is said that the child has taken after his mother or any other relative. Children can be overweight because of their genes, but this may not be true in all cases. In some cases the parents may extremely thin, but the child may be the opposite.

Food habits of the child have an impact on his health. If the child doesn't participate in active sports and spends most of his time in front of computer or T.V., he tends to put on weight.

AN ANALYSIS OF DIFFERENT BEHAVIOUR

If we analyse the different types of behaviour and habits in a child, the following salient points emerge:

- Upbringing of the child is of utmost importance –
- It is necessary that the child be made aware of "right" and "wrong" from his childhood.

- Do not dismiss the wrong habits of the child attributing them to his genes.
- Give a proper direction to the child's speech, behaviour and habits from his childhood itself.
- Proper food habits should be cultivated in the family. Give your child the food in adequate quantity at the appropriate time. Include milk, curd, green vegetables, fruits and such other healthy items in his meal to develop his immunity system. If the child is choosy about their food in his initial years, it can adversely impact his health in the long run. It is the responsibility of the parents to ensure that the child is given healthy and nutritious things in his meal.

3

EMOTIONAL PROBLEMS OF CHILDREN

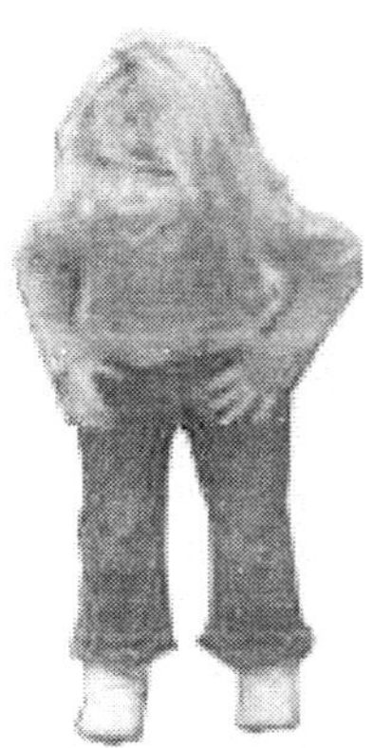

Children become victim of some emotional problems because of which they start behaving in an adverse manner. For example, a very intelligent child starts getting poor marks in the class or a very calm child suddenly starts becoming short-tempered and biting his nails. A child behaves in this manner only when he starts feeling emotionally insecure. There might be many reasons for this. For example, with the birth of younger brother or sister the division of the affection of the child, Father's going away from the family for a long period due to some work etc. Sometimes there is negligence towards the emotional and sensitive desires of the child during his upbringing, which gives rise to behavioural problems.

Children are naturally different from each other in terms of complexion, body and behaviour. If you happen to visit the nursery (new-born wing) in a hospital you can see that some of these young ones are active, some are dull, some of them are always crying while some are quiet. These are natural differences. These differences go passed on even as they grow up.

All of us are surrounded by internal confrontations.

Sometimes the subconscious self says something else while performing a duty or thinking about it. These confrontations don't allow a person to differentiate between right and wrong. Similar things happen in the lives of the children as well. Thereafter the mental dilemma is expressed in physical or emotional problems. Headache or stomach-ache, vertigo, unconsciousness, hysteria etc. can be the physical manifestations of the same.

Behaviour can change due to emotional problems. Different types of behaviour can be seen at different ages. Poor behaviour of the child should be not neglected and one should consult a Child Guidance Clinic to seek a solution for the problem.

• Till four years of age

The child must be taken for a check up if the following changes are seen in him over a period of time–severe restlessness, unresponsiveness, disinterestedness in having meals or milk and vomits after intakes, is always scared, is unable to go for his natural calls, and feels hesitant to talking to other children.

• Between four to eight years of age

One should be attentive if the child starts behaving in these manners due to emotional problems between four to eight years of age – the child does not play with the children of his age, starts fighting with them or sits away from them, always sticks to his mother, is unwilling to do any work, starts shouting or yelling without any reason, starts wetting his bed, feels scared of different things (like animals, darkness), is of destructive nature and breaks things, complains of stomach-ache, vomiting sensation before going to school, continues to suck his thumb etc.

- **Between eight and twelve years of age**

Children become mature by the time they reach this age and start participating and contributing in a number of activities both in the house and at school. The child has formed his own likes and dislikes by this time. But parents should start paying more attention to him when they notice behavioural and emotional changes in the child such as – if the child has become lethargic and just wants to keep sleeping or if he repeatedly keeps saying that no one loves him etc., is being disrespectful towards his parents and other elders at home, is losing interest in studies, is showing an inclination towards sex or appears lost.

- **Between twelve and fifteen years of age**

This period can be termed as the beginning of adolescence. Children undergo many physical and emotional changes during this age. Thus it becomes quite an unnerving and difficult task to expect children to act according to your wishes at this age. But the changes which should invite the attention of parents are – Biting the nails fervently, inability to make friends, not listening to teachers and parents, lagging behind in studies, a feeling of fear or nervousness over "growing up".

SOLUTIONS

Solutions can be easily found for these day-to-day problems of children. A well-meaning teacher, your family physician and an elderly person at home (grandparents) can prove to be a great help in this regard.

Specialists can be consulted for certain problems as well who can be – a speech therapist, consultants of a Child Guidance Clinic, Psychologists, Psychiatrists, and Social Workers etc. Child Guidance Clinics offer psychological and logical solutions to both parents and children and guide the children in the right direction. Parents can be counselled separately at different times for better effect.

Therapists try to understand the complete background (family situation, habits and relatives) of the child in order to get the root of the problem. Thereafter they successfully establish smooth relations and understanding between parents and the children. The natural strength of the child can be developed further by the treatment of the therapist so that the child feels self-confident all over again.

Apart from private physicians and child counselling clinics, the Ministry of Health has established a Child Guidance Clinic in New Delhi, which can be consulted for a number of problems pertaining to children. The address of the same is:

Child Guidance Clinic

College of Nursing (Near Vikram Hotel),

Lajpat Nagar-4, New Delhi – 110024

Ph: 26436668

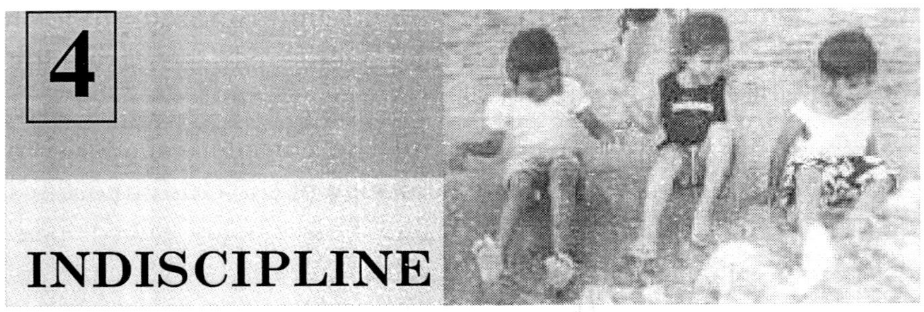

4 INDISCIPLINE

Born in a family after years of prayers for a child, Pintoo was a much pampered child. His whims and fancies were fulfilled even before they were uttered, being the only child in the family after years of yearning. He was the object of affection and attention of the elders and the young in the family. But despite all this, Pintoo was a disobedient child.

Once it happened that Pintoo was trying out to reach out to a box containing expensive crockery. His mother kept pleading with him not to play with such a thing, but her words fell on deaf ears and ultimately the box fell down. The entire crockery set was in pieces. Before Pintoo's mother could take him to task for this, her father-in-law intervened saying that it is in the element of children to be naughty at this age. There were many such instances when one person or the other came in the way of disciplining Pintoo whenever he did something unwanted.

Thus it became a habit for Pintoo to throw a tantrum if any of his demands were not fulfilled. This is a problem that many parents face with their children. If parents ignore these tantrums initially and fulfil their wrong demands then such children become completely undisciplined and disobedient when they grow up and turn into a cause of concern for their parents.

What exactly is Discipline?

In brief, respecting ones elders, understanding one's responsibility, following the path of truth, understanding others' needs and wishes can be termed as discipline. By means of discipline children can be taught and trained into acquiring habits that are considered appreciable by our society. Later on, following this very path can lead the child to success.

The following acts are considered to be acts of indiscipline: obstinacy, disobedience, being stubborn, arguing with elders, answering back, not listening to elders, Being disrespectful towards elders, being selfish (not sharing with brothers/sisters/ friends), being violent with other children without any reason, spitting on others, use of slippers/shoes etc. to hit others, fighting with sibling reason, beating classmates and pulling hair.

Every society and family is governed by some rules. A disciplined child understands and perceives those rules according to his age and behaves accordingly. The child learns all these things from his family members and the surrounding atmosphere. Even an infant or a toddler can very well differentiate between appreciation, scolding, and punishment by the tone of the person. On being reprimanded on doing something wrong, the child comes to understand that behaviour as unacceptable behaviour.

We have to bear it in mind that no child learns discipline on his own. It is largely upto the methodology used by the parents to discipline the child that he learns to differentiate right from the wrong and then child goes a long way in fulfilling his duties and responsibilities effectively as he grows up.

Discipline to what extent?

A child has to be taught discipline keeping in mind his age and accordingly he should be given freedom as well. Discipline is no sense means curtailing or curbing the freedom of a child.

In fact effective discipline is establishing a co-ordination between independence and discipline.

However, if the child is given more freedom than he can handle, he finds himself surrounded in a helpless situation. For instance, if your 5 year old son/daughter throws a tantrum that she wants to drive your car and you decide to pacify her/him by making her/him sit in your lap while you drive. You may think that you have done an extremely wise thing, but in reality you are committing a big mistake as you are teaching your child to be undisciplined. By doing this, you are inviting the child to throw a fit to sit at the steering wheel every time you drive and secondly you are diverting your own attention too. On the one hand you are violating traffic rules and on the other hand, by giving in to her wrong demands you are making him obstinate.

Can a child be given the permission to swim if he doesn't know how to swim? We have to understand that giving the child adequate opportunity to fulfil both his social and physical requirements is the basic requirement of discipline. Every child knows the distinction between his reasonable and unreasonable demands from within. He also knows the extent to which his demands will be fulfilled. If the child is reprimanded for a wrong action of his, even though he shows an outward protest for the same, actually he has an innate requirement to be disciplined by his parents. Many undisciplined children on seeing or interacting with disciplined children too wish their parents had given them a right disciplined upbringing.

If you scold or taunt a child at every step, he is bound to become self-centred and obstinate. This way he will only think about fulfilling his wishes and not listen to his elders. Over discipline or control does no good to the child. A child should be guided on the basis of their age, situation and specific context if any.

Good discipline lays the foundation for a healthy and

balanced personality. Excessive strictness and discipline can prove to be harmful. Suppose a very small child snatches something from your hand and it happens to slip from his hand and break: If you begin hitting the child now in the name of disciplining him, it would hardly discipline him and you too will unnecessarily spoil your image in front of the people who are present.

Over discipline often renders a child submissive. It hampers his development and chances are that he will become rebellious and naughty. Therefore make sure you discipline the child in a balanced manner.

POSSIBLE CAUSES OF INDISCIPLINE

Just as the old maxim goes, "Rome was not built in a day', similarly any child (whether big or small) doesn't become undisciplined in a day. This happens over a period of time. As we have discussed in the earlier chapters as well, every child has an innate capacity to understand certain rules from the infant stage itself. Even through the medium of crying children can communicate various situations/emotions such as hunger, loneliness, longing for the mother's attention etc. When others begin to fulfil their unsaid demands because of their crying, they begin to understand that they can get their demands fulfilled by crying. The following may be the possible reasons behind a child's undisciplined behaviour :

- **Giving too much liberty and independence to the children**

Some parents (more so of today's modern age) pride themselves in calling themselves liberal and giving complete independence to their children. Such parents avoid saying anything to curb their children. These children naturally become very self- centred and only act according to their fancies. Gradually they just want to be left on their own. This stage begins to cause bother and worry the parents. The children go out of their control completely and even teachers start reporting the indiscipline of the children to the parents.

- **Very strict behaviour/upbringing**

If children are not given liberty to do anything according to their will and are constantly terrorized by parents, they start ignoring what their parents say. Such children then do not give respect to their elders and start moving into the category of undisciplined children. For example, if your child wants to go out and play and you hold him up strictly asking him to study. You do not let him go out even after he has finished his homework/portion etc. This will give a sense of disappointment to the child and even though he will be sitting with his books, his mind would be on playing. Given an opportunity, he will put his books aside and run out to play.

If your child wishes to buy something, which is also well within your reach, denying him the thing on the pretext of controlling and disciplining him will only make rebellious and undisciplined later.

- **Excessive pampering and love or non-uniform love**

Certain families over indulge in their children in terms of pampering or loving their children beyond the reasonable limits. Children on their own, invite love and affection from the known and the unknown alike. But letting the child away for bad behaviour, mischief or misdeed in the name of love is unacceptable as this way the child is shown the path to indiscipline by his own family. Not scolding the child or correcting him for any form of wrong or unacceptable behaviour will also confuse the child between right and wrong. In families with two or more children, it is common to see one child (by virtue or his being younger, elder or any other reason) being loved and pampered more. Normally parents and other family members tend to spoil this child more and make him obstinate and undisciplined.

Anu's son Sabir was loved and pampered by everyone in the family. The pampering was in such extremes that grandparents, uncle and aunt never let Anu reprimand or correct Sabir even if committed mischief or misbehaved with anyone. As time passed Sabir became a much undisciplined child. After a few years Anu was blessed with another male child. But by that time Sabir had become so spoilt and uncompromising that he refused to share anything with his younger brother Kabir. He used to snatch anything that made his brother happy and Kabir was left crying.

In a similar fashion some children learn abusive language because of too much love and pampering. When initially children use bad words, parents and elders start laughing out of astonishment and amusement. Children take this as an encouragement and adopt bad words as a part of their daily language.

- **An attempt to make your child extremely obedient**

As parents if you expect your child to be obedient all the time; eat, sleep, study etc. when you ask him to, then he will become rebellious at one point or the other in order to fulfil his wishes. In such a situation discipline becomes a problem in itself. It is not possible to control each and every action of the child according to your wishes.

- **An atmosphere of discord in the house**

Children who come from families which have an unpleasant and disorganised atmosphere are generally seen to be highly undisciplined. If the child sees his elders arguing, fighting or taunting each other, they too imbibe these values very easily. If the family members nest negative feelings such as envy among each other and are not on friendly terms, the children in the family too learn such negative feelings by observing their elders. The children are always exposed to different arguments and unpleasant situations and are unable to differentiate the right from the wrong.

In joint families it is not uncommon to find feelings of jealousy, conspiracy etc. because of different financial levels among brothers etc. Children are witness to these things and they too keep imbibing these very things in their conscience and learn gossiping, backbiting, foul language and such other negative qualities quite easily.

- **Lack of adequate space**

Children need proper space for rest and playing both in the house and outside. Sometimes houses are so small and compact that it is not possible to keep expensive decorative pieces put of their reach. In this situation children need to be constantly curbed and controlled to avoid accidents which sometimes become a hindrance in the path of disciplining them. The child begins to become obstinate and rebellious because of constant nagging and scolding and continues to play in the place where he is prohibited.

- **Unstable and confused mindset of the parents**

If parents behave differently with children in the same set of situations, then child gets confused between right and wrong. Let us understand this statement through these examples. Suppose there is a wall or tree next to your house which your child loves to climb. Generally, you consciously or unconsciously do not pay attention to this action. But in front of guests and relatives you start shouting at your child for the same. Similarly you have prohibited your child from eating the ice cream from the local vendor. But you give in at times when she/he throws a tantrum instead of standing by your instruction. At other times however, when you are in a disciplining mood you start getting extremely stringent with your child. Contradictory reactions of parents in both the above examples completely put the child in a baffled state about what he can and can't do.

The bottom-line is when you wish to prohibit your child from doing something, stick to your words. Do not falter between leniency and strictness. Your inability to stand by your words will encourage your child to become disrespectful towards you.

- **The feeling of panic when the child starts crying**

Some parents panic when the child starts crying. It is normal for children to start crying when they see their demands are not being fulfilled. Parents do not know what to do in such a situation. They feel completely helpless as the child starts crying louder and louder. Finally they succumb to the child. Now as the child grows older and more observant, he understands that his crying is a weakness for his parents. Whenever he sees the situation becoming unfavourable for him, he resorts to crying as he knows that his parents will fulfil his demand eventually. He thus becomes obstinate and undisciplined.

Even if parents are strict, there may be others in the family such as grandparents who want to fulfil everything that the child demands. They become a shield for the child even he is being unreasonable and naughty. In this situation parents become completely helpless. The child understands the situation and tries to use it to his advantage whenever he gets an opportunity. He begins to get used to "yes' all the time. Even in outdoor situations he uses his crying as a weapon to get what he wants.

Some children scream loudly, some cry, while some others bang their heads on the walls to get their demands fulfilled. All these come under negative behaviour. If parents let their child go on like this unchecked, all these become permanent traits for him. It is therefore up to the parents to prevent their child from becoming obstinate. Initial negligence can cause a lot of problem later.

- **Attention seeking behaviour**

Some children display undisciplined behaviour to seek the attention of family members. If they feel that the elders are busy in their own activities and are not paying any need to him, they start indulging in activities such as screaming, throwing things around or crying loudly. Thus they get used to such behaviour showing indiscipline.

HOW CAN WE DISCIPLINE OUR CHILDREN?

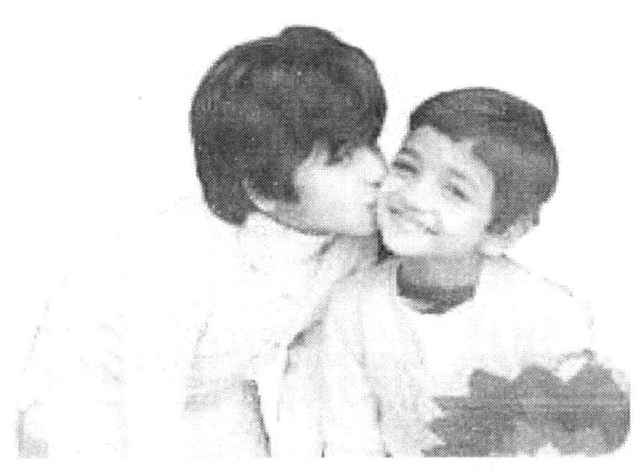

Making the child agree to something forcibly is not called discipline. He should be properly guided into right behaviour from his initial years. In addition to this parents should also pay attention to the following things as well:

- Children should be made to realise the benefits of mixing up with other children and family members. This will also ensure a peaceful atmosphere at home.

- Do not make an attempt to forcibly ask the child to act in a certain manner. Do not criticise or scold the child over and over again for a wrong action or behaviour. Instead praise and acknowledge his right efforts. Scold or be strict when you feel it is necessary in the direction of teaching correct discipline to the child.
- Parents should be aware of the growing needs of the children as they grow, else the children can resort to wrong habits to fulfil their needs. For example, as the child turns two-three years of age, he feels an urge to scribble with a pencil or pen. Therefore, in this stage he can be given a pencil and notebook or chalk and slate or a small blackboard. This way he will not scribble on walls and other places.
- Do not embrace the child by taunting him again and again for any wrong action. This would only give rise to anger and resentment in him.
- Create an open and friendly atmosphere at home for your child to discuss debate and approach you for his queries and inquisitiveness. This will enable him to overcome his shyness and disappointment over "non-open' issues.
- Do not suppress his internal rebelliousness. Give him an opportunity to express his feelings and inner emotions.
- There should be a fixed direction to discipline. Be firm in "yes' or "no'. Do not say "No' to something today only to give in to his pressure and agree to the same later.
- Parents should never discipline their children to vent out their anger or disappointment.
- Be disciplined and organised yourself. This will be a live model for your child to emulate and follow.
- Do not resort to lecturing your child between "right',

"wrong", "cause' and "effect' of behaviour. His mind is not developed enough to be able to realise and understand such things in detail.

- Inculcate good habits and right behavior in the child from his initial years. Never succumb to his tantrums and accept anything that you think is inappropriate for him. If you yield to his demands if he cries, rolls on the floor or with any such action, your child will always use these actions to blackmail you in the future as well.
- Loving your child definitely does not mean that you accept everything he says or does whether right or wrong. Control and discipline him as and when he need for the same arises.
- In case of two or more children, make sure that you treat all children uniformly. Partiality or "favouritism" towards one can create inferiority complex in the other which can create complications and problems for all children in the future.
- The child should be taught/given an opportunity to learn things according to his age and capacity. Over independence or over restriction often makes the children undisciplined.
- Discipline should be stable and uniform. The child should be clearly told the "Dos' and Don'ts". If the child is wise enough, explain to him why he shouldn't do a certain thing or why a certain action is wrong. He should know that he can be punished if he does a prohibited action. If there is a difference of opinion between the parents over an issue, they should sort it out later. If parents argue or disagree in front of the children, children become disobedient.
- While disciplining the child, it is very important that parents do not interfere with each other's instructions. One parent should avoid supporting the child while he is being scolded for a wrong action by the other parent.

- A small example to illustrate the above would be sufficient if a father asks his daughter to change her dress and shoes before going out to play and the mother opposes the father saying that uniform is fine and needn't be changed as it is to be washed the next day.
- If the parents of the child don't get along well and arguments and disagreements go on a regular basis, then they often find faults with each other's disciplinary behaviour. This way the child loses respect for his elders and takes advantage of the situation. Lack of harmony between parents can also become a cause for indiscipline.
- Do not compare your child with his friend or his sibling. Comparison instills a feeling of inferiority in the child and he begins to build anger and resentfulness against the other child. Because of this he starts displaying an undisciplined behaviour.

Punishments for Indiscipline

It sometimes becomes unavoidable to punish the child for indiscipline. However punishments are best avoided. As far as possible try to make do with verbally chastising him or making him understand affectionately. The purpose of punishment should be to rectify the wrong behaviour of the children and not to take revenge from the child on any account. The whole purpose of punishment is to curb any form of social or behavioural anomalies. Punishment and discipline are complicated issues. Appreciation and rewards are a better mode of disciplining the child on any given day. However, sometimes it becomes impossible to discipline without punishment. If the child repeatedly commits the same prohibited action, then punishment can make him deter from the same. Punishment can be in the form of a beating, isolating the child in a room or prohibiting against using a certain thing (like T.V., games) etc. It is however very important to keep in mind the following things while punishing the child:

- After awarding a punishment on doing a wrong thing, keep the atmosphere of the house normal and calm. Do not prolong the punishment and do not repeatedly remind him of his mistake.
- Punishment should be in accordance with the gravity of his mistake and his age.
- The child should clearly understand the purpose of this punishment. Do not discuss the situation again and again after telling the reason once. For example, 6 year old Sonu used to pinch or scratch his baby sister at any given opportunity. His mother's repeated requests and threats had no effect on him. So one day she gave him a punishment which was that for 2 days he was totally forbidden to enter the baby's room, leave alone see her or play with her. It took only one day for Sonu to realise his mistake after which he went to his mother and apologised for his mistake. Then he immediately ran off to pick up the baby and play with her.
- As far as possible, punish the child at the time when he commits the mistake. Punishing the child hours later has no meaning. For instance, your child wants to eat his breakfast without brushing his teeth, while you are insisting on brushing his teeth first. The child keeps standing adamantly and the others members have started their breakfast. You give in to him and ask him to join others. Hours later you starts taunting or scolding him for his obstinate behaviour during morning hours. This is completely wrong and useless. If you wish to discipline the child in the right way, then punish him at the time of mistake, not later.
- It is best to ignore an unconscious mistake/wrong action or behaviour. If he repeats the mistake, punish him again in a similar manner. Do not forgive him or let him go the next time he commits the mistake again.

- The punishment should be according to his mistake and if possible, related to the mistake. For instance, if the child has spilled or thrown food/milk, he should be asked to wipe the mess and not refused the meal altogether.
- Never resort to severe or very strict punishments. If you raise your hand at the child at each and every mistake he will become completely stubborn and no amount of punishment would have any effect on him. Such children know that for whatever mistake they do, the maximum punishment would be a beating etc. So they tend to become indifferent towards any warning or punishment and in fact become even more undisciplined when punished. They dismiss and avoid what elders say to them to rectify them.

FOR TEACHERS

Generally children start becoming undisciplined from the age of 2-3 years, for which the responsibility largely rests with parents or other family members. However, in some cases children learn indiscipline at school as well, which they believe to be mischief or naughtiness. When such behaviour becomes a habit, children start behaving in the same way in front of their teachers as well.

It is also the responsibility of the teachers to try to bring about an improvement in the children. If the child bullies or hits other children, spits etc. then the teacher should try to find out the reason behind his behaviour. The teacher should also study and analyse the behaviour of his friends and classmates etc. As far as possible the teacher should try to make the child understand softly; however he/she can also take recourse to mild punishments if necessary. To discipline young and adolescent children, one should adopt a behaviour according to their age and punish them too accordingly if necessary.

☸ ☸

5

FOOD AVOIDING TENDENCIES IN CHILDREN

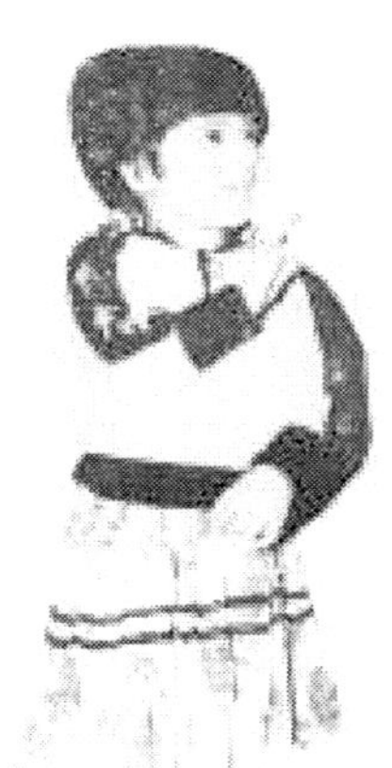

It is a very common sight in households to see mothers following children with a plate of food in their hands. The child is busy in his play or T.V. and the mother just about manages to put in a bite into his mouth when the child runs off again. The mother keeps following the child telling him anecdotes and stories to make him eat. In this whole process the mother is unable to concentrate on her food because the child feeding process is so time consuming that by the time he finishes his meal, she has lost all her interest in it. Low appetite and lack of interest in having food becomes a major cause of worry for the mothers. If the child is forcibly fed, he vomits the entire food, which makes forcible feeding too a wasteful exercise.

I approached child specialist Dr. Sonika Aggarwal to suggest remedies for this omnipresent problem, who gave me the following measures during the course of our discussion:

- Never feed the child forcibly and do not offer him enticements such as chocolate, toffee etc. to make him eat. This will complicate the problem more rather than rectifying it.

- Never scare or terrorise the child into having food. For example, never tell him that a crow, ghost etc. would come if he/she doesn't eat and so on.
- Children divert their minds to other things very soon. This is more so in the case of children who show allergy towards food. Such children either start paying attention to T.V. or start looking at things on the road etc. Therefore, try and give food to the child in a room which doesn't have such distractions. Also do not switch on T.V. during his meal time.
- Do not display your worry anger overtly if the child doesn't eat. Children throw more tantrums when they see your anger or frustration. Remove the plate quietly if the child continues to avoid eating and pretend that it's absolutely alright if he doesn't eat. This might seem difficult initially but this can solve the problem.
- Try and fix a 'meal time' for the family so that the entire family can sit down to have food, while sharing their experiences and laughter. Also make the child sit at the dining table with the family. Try and get colourful (with cartoon motifs etc.) and attractive table mats, spoons, forks etc., so that the child gets attracted towards food as well.
- Show your love and appreciation for the child with a hug or a kiss after he finishes his entire meal. You can also give him a small token when he finishes his food. It is preferable to give him a story or a game (session with you) as a prize instead of material things.
- Fix a proper time for the child's breakfast, lunch and dinner. Also avoid stuffing him with too much snacks such as chips, wafers, chocolates, soft drinks during the meal intervals as it will fill his stomach and will not leave much space for food.

- If the child is not taking food, then do not give in to his demands of biscuits, sweets etc. thinking that at least he is having those. This way the child will get used to filling his stomach with these things and will never develop a craving for food.
- If the child expresses a desire to have food with his own hands let him do so. Do not worry over petty issues like his spilling food or mixing up food and eating in a messy way. Even if he wants to enjoy his meal as a game, let him.
- Do not habituate the child to take soft drinks, chips etc. just before meal time.
- Some children have a tendency to eat slowly. If your child eats slowly, then do not force him to eat quickly. However pay equal attention to the fact that the child doesn't get distracted in T.V. or games etc. while eating. Allot a maximum time slot of half an hour to the child to finish his meal.
- Do not ask the child his preferences in food at the time when he sits down to eat. Let him eat whatever has been prepared at that time. In case of a new dish, introduce him to the dish with everyone at the table.
- Do not give the child too much food at one time. Give him small portions of food, subsequently giving him more when he finishes one portion. If the child refuses to eat the food at that time, do not remove his plate and offer him an alternative option.
- If the child tells you that his stomach is full, then do not make an effort to give him more food by telling him jokes etc. In such a situation the child might get irritated and throw off the plate, vomit or cry out loudly to express his anger and frustration.

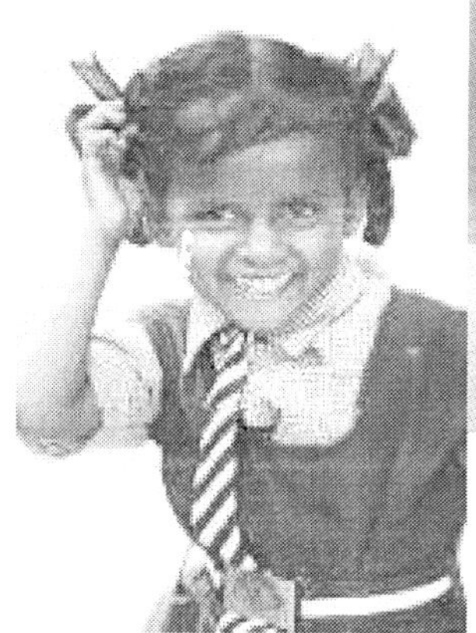

6

THE PROBLEM OF BED-WETTING

Five-year old Kanu started bed wetting (passing urine in the bed while sleeping) all of a sudden which startled her mother Priya. Priya had toilet-trained Kanu from the age of six months itself and this was possibly the first time Kanu had done such a thing ever since. The first time this happened Priya thought that Kanu must have been extremely frightened about something because of which she had wet the bed. In the morning when Kanu woke up Priya started asking her why she had done such a thing. But Kanu kept mum despite being questioned again and again, Priya got exasperated and gave Kanu a slap with the warning of never to do such a thing in the future.

But the following afternoon Kanu repeated the same action and started weeping aloud. Despite being scolded by Priya again Kanu continued to wet her bed on consecutive days as well. Priya was in complete darkness about the new development in Kanu and she realised that her cajoling and scolding alike were not having any effect on Kanu. Finally Priya, on the advice of her husband decided to consult a child physician for the problem. When they explained the complete scenario before him; he simply smiled and said "Kanu is completely fine. She doesn't have a medical problem at all. Infact this young one

(Kanu's little brother) is the reason behind Kanu's problem". As the physician pointed towards the infant in Priya's hands, both Priya and her husband were astonished. The physician saw the expression on their faces and explained with a smile, "See, in simple words I can tell you that Kanu has developed a tendency of jealousy against her brother. She must have felt that your attention has been diverted from her on the arrival of the new baby. Hence, she has started bed wetting to draw your attention back to her again. If you pay attention to her and shower her with love and affection, she will be normal soon."

The physician was absolutely right. As Priya and her husband heeded his advice and gave Kanu equal attention in the coming days, she was soon back to her earlier active, cheerful self.

There can be many reasons like the above one for the problem of bed wetting of 4-5 year olds. There are behavioural as well as physical causes behind this problem. These days modern educated parents cultivate proper toilet habits in the children right from the infant stage. Children too respond to toilet training at the initial stages well and soon they themselves start giving indications when nature calls. Sometimes during the chilly winter days 2-3 year old children pass urine in the bed, which can be taken as an exception. But when older children of 8-9 years start bed wetting, it definitely has a serious reason behind it.

CAUSES

There can be many psychological and physical reasons behind bed wetting. Child specialist, Dr. Jyoti Agrawal enumerates the following causes:

- If the child's stomach has been infected by worms,

sometimes he finds it difficult to control his urinary bladder. He passes urine unconsciously in the bed in such a situation.

- During the teething process children tend to pass urine more often, which is more pronounced in the night as compared to the day. Then the child tends to wet his bed.
- Some children are unable to exercise control over their bladder because of which the child passes urine without his own knowledge.
- If the child suffers from constipation, even then he can have the problem of bed wetting.
- If the child is extremely weak, he cannot control all his physical actions completely. In such a situation the child feels weak and lax and wets his bed.
- If the PH of the child's urine is more acidic, and the child has irritation around his private organs, (which can be indicative of an infection) and therefore he tends to wet his bed.
- If the child is very coward, he fears at night with darkness, believes in ghosts, he is likely to wet his bed at night even at the age of 7 or 8 years.

PSYCHOLOGICAL AND BEHAVIOURAL CAUSES

- **Deep seated fear about something**

Eight year old Samir started wetting his bed suddenly. His parents started reprimanding him, but it yielded no effect. Finally Samir's father sat down with him one day and asked him affectionately. Initially Samir hesitated, but his father's persistent cajoling made him open finally.

Samir explained to his father that in the night he feels

extremely scared to go out of his room. Now this fear, as his father found out, had been framed in his heart because one of his classmates had been telling horror stories and ghost tales in the class. The boy had narrated certain incidents wherein he had said that if a ghost caught a human being, he would torture the person very badly.

These tales and narration had left such a deep impression in Samir's heart that he was too scared to leave his room even if he had to go to the toilet. Therefore he used to suppress his urge to use the toilet and then he had wet his bed.

Thus in this manner if any type of fear captures a child then he starts wetting his bed unconsciously. Fear can be of the following types:

1. If the child has been severely reprimanded or beaten for a mistake, which has completely terrified him, he acquires great fear for such punishments.
2. If the child is particularly scared of a teacher or a relative etc. at home.
3. If the child fears darkness.
4. The child is terrified of ghosts, spirits etc.
5. If the child is scared of desolate, isolated places.
6. If the child has been strictly instructed to complete a certain work else face punishments and in case he fails to complete it by the stipulated time, he feels scared to face the next day.

- **The feeling of jealousy or insecurity**

If the child has a feeling of jealousy or insecurity within, then his digestive process is influenced as well. These processes aggravate the acidity in the body, which is flushed out of the body in the form of urine.

The feeling of jealously or insecurity can stem in the child by a yet to arrive or an already arrived new one. If the elder child is gripped by any of the above feelings because parents are unable to pay him the attention he was used to earlier, then he can start bedwetting.

- **Dreams**

Some children get so engrossed in a fascinating dream that they lose control over their body at that time. Consequently they are unable to control their bladder at that time and end up wetting the bed.

Similarly some children get so frightened by a bad dream that they wet their bed. However this can be exceptional as children wet the bed under the influence of dreams do not tend to repeat this time and again.

- **Lack of adequate training**

Normally children should be given toilet training right from the infant stage itself. If this stage has been ignored by the parents, then the children tend to be careless and oblivious to their toilet instincts even as they grow up. Such types of children have a tendency to wet their beds.

It is normally observed that the children of working mothers are with baby sitters/maids during most part of the day, they naturally do not pay much attention to cultivating good toilets habits in children. Mothers have less time at their disposal with the children because of their working hours. In the evenings fatigue and impending household work beckon her attention. When the child voices his urge to urinate or to do potty, the harried mother asks the child to look into it himself or go to the bathroom to relieve himself, instead of teaching/ training the child herself. Such children keep bedwetting every now and then.

Such a situation can arise during the night time as well. If the child gets up in the middle of the night and tells his mother that he wants to go the toilet, instead of taking him then, if she pats him to sleep, he is bound to wet the bed later.

- **Unfamiliar surroundings**

If the child has to sleep in an unfamiliar place at some time, then his discomfort in the new place or his nervousness can make him wet his bed there even if he has not been normally doing thus at home. This can happen at a relative's place or in a hotel (during a vacation) etc.

- **Carelessness on the mother's part**

Some mothers are careless by nature and never pay any attention to their children's mischief or to their toilet habits. Even if their fairly grown up child is not conscious about his toilet habits, they laugh and ignore the matter altogether. On the other hand, such mothers are deeply offended if someone else tries to counsel them of their children on this issue. They try to defend their children's wrong habits by being loud in their dissent. Thereafter they offer to clean up the mess wishing to finish the matter. Such children are prone to wet the bed as well.

- **Extremely talkative or busy mother**

Rajni lived with her three year old son Rajat and her

husband in a joint family. She and the other ladies of the family were always engaged in some or the other work in order to fulfil the demands of the family. Rajat was brought up with utmost love and affection by the elders in the family. Rajni herself had never realised how Rajat has turned three years of age. But there was one habit of Rajat that greatly bothered Rajni and her husband. Rajat used to call his mother whenever he felt an urge to use the toilet but before she could rush to him he used to relieve himself wherever he was – in kitchen, bathroom or living room. The elders in the family used to scold him but Rajat was totally unaffected by it. Rajat was to be given admission in a school shortly, so this habit if his was causing a lot of distress to his parents.

Once an elder relative happened to pay them a visit. She too happened to observe the situation at Rajni's house and call Rajni to talk to her. Rajni immediately started defending herself saying that Rajat never waited for her to come and take him to the bathroom. But the old aunt would have none of it. She had observed that Rajni would be so engrossed in her work or talking to other ladies that she would take 6-7 minutes to go to Rajat even after he had called her many times. She told Rajni that she should habituate Rajat to use the toilet by taking him to the toilet herself after specific intervals of time. Gradually this training would make Rajat give up his habit of relieving himself anywhere and everywhere.

Thus when ladies are too busy talking or doing their work and do not respond to their children's call of going to the bathroom, the children slowly develop a tendency to ignore their own urges. Such children are also prone to be victims of the problem of bedwetting.

- **Attention seeking behaviour**

If the child has not been getting due attention at his school and home despite his putting his best efforts in studies, art, regularity etc., he begins to build frustration and anger within him, which finds an outlet through his bedwetting.

Also, as I explained earlier, if his younger brother/sister has been demanding more time and attention of his parents and this child has been feeling lonely and ignored, then also he starts wetting his bed to draw the attention of his parents to himself.

Four year old Gagan wet his bed in the night once. On being questioned by his mother in the morning, he started crying and then said complainingly, "You never scold Isha when she does the same in your lap." His mother understood his complex. She took Gagan in her arms and explained lovingly, "Gagan, Isha is very small. She neither talks nor walks. But you are a smart boy. When she too grows up like you, she will also not do such things." Gagan was convinced and never wet his bed again.

MEASURES TO TACKLE THE PROBLEM

If your child is suffering from this problem, then it is not a very difficult task to overcome the problem. Paying attention to small things and changing some habits of the child can easily help you get rid of the problem. If the child has a physical problem, take him to a doctor so that he can treat the child.

The following steps can be taken if the child is wetting the bed because of psychological and behavioural problems:

- Even if you are engaged in some work or are exhausted, you should pay immediate attention to the child's call to go to the toilet. Similarly during the night if the child wishes to be taken to the toilet, instead of scolding him and putting him to sleep, the mother should take him to the toilet and then put him back to sleep.

- If the child wakes you during deep sleep for taking him to the toilet and you scold him or clearly express your irritation etc., the child might get scared and refuse to relieve himself in the bathroom. In this situation he will wet his bed in his sleep. Never scold him whenever he tells his urge.
- Try and avoid giving him lot of water to drink during the night time. Make this up by giving him adequate fluids and water during the day time. Give him enough water during the day time. Give him enough water after his meals. Take the child to the bathroom definitely before taking him to bed.
- Do not give the child warm beverages such as tea and coffee one hour before sleep time.
- Do not be harsh with the child when he wets his bed. Explain to him softly and patiently and lend a patient ear to his problems, else the child will develop an inferiority complex which will aggravate the problem more.
- See to it that you do not let the child be engulfed by feelings of jealousy, insecurity etc. If there has been new entrant (baby) in the family, pay adequate attention to the elder child as well. Do not neglect him at any cost. You have to understand the elder child understands love and security much better than the young one. Do not make the elder one feel that he has been deprived of the love and affection of his parents after the coming of the young one. Pay more attention to him if possible.
- Small children tend to pass more urine during winters because of the cold. Make arrangements to keep the child warm during winters. Warm the child's bed by laying soft blankets underneath the bedsheet or by keeping warm water bottles on the bed at a safe distance from the child.

Heat convector, air conditioners etc. can also be used to increase the room temperature. Never sleep with these electrical appliances on. Switch them off before going to sleep. If the child is kept adequately warm, then he will not have an urge to pass urine time and again.

- If the child is in infant stage, he should first be tightly wrapped in a shawl or blanket and then a quilt should be covered on him. This way even if he pushes off the quilt by moving his legs, he would still be warm from within and will not pass urine frequently.
- Do not make the child sleep in front of the cooler during the rainy weather.
- As a rule make the child use the bathroom while he is sleeping every 2-2½ hours irrespective of the weather. Also children generally go to bed earlier than the parents. Make them go to the bathroom before putting them to sleep.
- Parents and teachers should keep building the child's self-confidence. Always appreciate him when he does a good job.
- Start toilet training the child from his infant stage. If you habituate the infant by taking him to the toilet every one hour or so, he will understand that he is not to wet his nappy. Soon he will start giving you indications like whimpering etc. whenever he feels the urge to pass urine. You will be surprised to know even 2-3 month old infant is capable of giving such indications. As the child grows up, he will subsequently know that he should go to the bathroom to relieve himself. Such children will never relieve themselves just about anywhere (including the bed). Right training by the mother will always make the child learn to do things at the right time and at the right place.

- Do not let the child cultivate any type of fear in his psyche – of darkness, ghosts or any other fear. Clear and eliminate his fears by rationally explaining all such fears to be baseless.
- If the child continues to wet his bed despite observing all the above measures, then carry out his urine examination and give him proper medication on the doctor's advice.
- If the child is suffering from incontinence (inability to control this bladder), then take medicines to strengthen the bladder on the advice of the doctor. Homeopathy and Ayurveda streams of medicines have many remedies for this problem.
- If the child continues to wet his bed on a regular basis, then consult a doctor immediately. Seeing the condition of the child and by conducting various tests on the urine of the child the doctor can come to a right diagnosis. It is quite possible that the child has some internal weakness.
- After the child turns 5-6 years of age, it is beneficial to give him two dates before he retires to bed. If he refuses to have dates, he can be given 3-4 almonds instead.
- Proper guidance of the parents and impartial behaviour on the part of the teachers can be a major aid in curing this problem effectively.

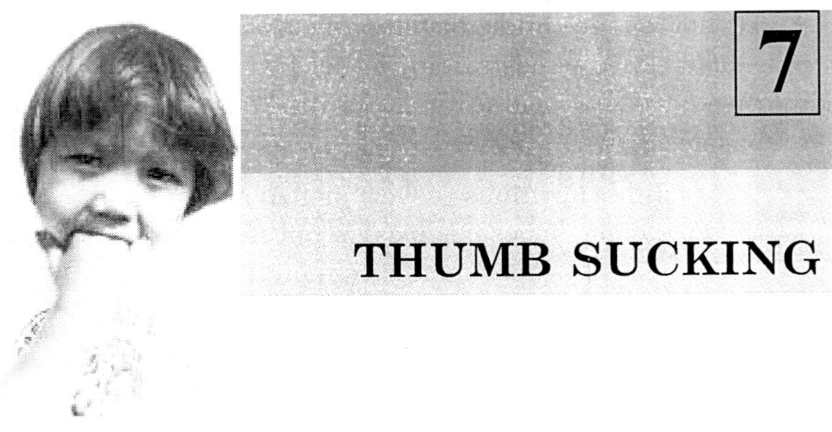

7 THUMB SUCKING

There are many lovable activities of small children like their radiant smile, their newly erupted front teeth, walking on their knees, sucking their thumb of hands or legs and many such activities which capture our attention immediately. At this time we will feel like picking them up and shower kisses and hugs on the child. Such activities attract the attention of not only of the kith and kin of the child but also of those who do not claim to be very good with kids.

Thumb sucking is an action which is acceptable in children till they are about one or one and a half years of age, after which it becomes an eyesore for the parents. Parents start looking for ways and means by which they can get their child get rid of this habit. But this is easier said than done. Once a child acquires the habit of thumb sucking, then it becomes very difficult for the child and parents alike to make him rid of this habit. The child immediately puts the other thumb inside his mouth the moment someone removes his thumb.

At this stage parents feel extremely helpless as no amount of their scolding or explaining has any effect on the child. Some children tend to suck two fingers together instead of the thumb. According to specialists, thumb sucking is a natural process.

Children have a tendency to suck their thumb right from their birth to about three years of age. Thumb sucking is in no way a symbol of physical weakness/anomaly.

In medical history there are varied opinions on the issue of the age till which thumb sucking can be considered normal. The age after which thumb sucking can be considered a problem too has divided opinions. Some doctors feel that the process of thumb sucking can be considered normal till the age of 4 years, while others feel that there is absolutely no need for parents to panic till the child is 6 years of age.

Thumb sucking is a normal activity in children and is seen in 70-80% of the children. But this comes down to about 30-35% as the children starts growing up. This comes down further to 14% till the children are 6 years of age, and is just about 5-6% for children more than 11 years.

NEGATIVE CONSEQUENCES OF THUMB SUCKING

Thumb sucking is a harmless activity. Nevertheless if the child continues to suck his thumb even after 5-6 years, it can have the following negative consequences:

- **Distortion in the shape of teeth and gums**

If a child continues to suck his thumb after 5-6 years also, then the shape of his teeth can get affected and his teeth might get distorted. If the child gets rid of this habit before his permanent teeth emerge then the teeth are not likely to be affected. Continuous thumb sucking can result in protruding teeth and disfiguration of jaws.

- **Unsymmetrical jaw**

Research conducted in America on the subject has proved that if a child continues to suck his thumb even after 5 years of age, he is likely to suffer from a disease in which one of the jaws becomes bigger or smaller than the other jaw. Thus the jaws appear unsymmetrical and the shape of the mouth and the face in totality appears completely distorted. These researchers have concluded that if the child is given a soother to suck, then the soother being soft, does not affect the shape of the jaws.

- **Bacterial infection**

Thumb sucking can result in the child contracting a bacterial infection because of continuous exposure to the thumb, which may be dirty many a times. This can cause a bacterial infection in the stomach and affect the digestion of the child.

- **Psychological pressure**

If a child has a habit of thumb sucking and the parents and other relatives of the child constantly chide the child for it, then it is likely to have an adverse effect on the child's psyche.

- **Peeling off the skin surface of the hand**

Some children suck their thumbs for such long intervals of time that the skin of their hands and the skin hair too starts getting peeled off, which starts hurting the child. At this time the child wishes to control his habit and this is the time when the child's parents should lend him a supporting hand.

- **Disfiguration of the thumb**

Continuous thumb sucking results in the thumb becoming thin and shrivelled and the consequent weakening of the thumb.

- **Speech defects**

Children who suck their thumbs often talk with their thumbs in their mouth. This results in wrong pronunciation of words and other subsequent speech defects. Their speech clarity is also compromised.

- **Injury in the mouth**

Excessive and repeated thumb sucking can even result in an injury in the mouth.

- **Distorted lips**

Thumb sucking for long intervals can result in swelling of the upper lip along with the protruding of the upper teeth which disfigures the face and the face begins to look abnormal and ugly.

POSSIBLE CAUSES OF THUMB SUCKING

Psychologists the world over believe that the thumb sucking activity pacifies the hunger and thirst in a child. Also it soothes the child. According to Dr. Patrick Freeman of Child Development Department, Philadelphia, thumb sucking inculcates the feeling of self-reliance in newborns and small children. Dr. Patrick observed during his research that when small children get hurt or fall sick, thumb sucking at this time relieves and soothes the children. However this activity starts appearing abnormal when children continue with it even as they grow older. At that time this activity can also have harmful effects on the child. The following can be the main causes for thumb sucking:

- **A source of relaxation and entertainment for the child**

Small children get into the habit of thumb sucking as it provides relaxation to the child. Dr. Patrick Freeman during his research came to this conclusion that children who breast feed often want to hold on to that feeling of security by sucking their thumb. When the child falls down during the time he is learning to walk then sucking the thumb soothes him and makes him forget his pain.

- **Nuclear family setup**

These days' Nuclear family setups are found generally where the mothers have multiple responsibilities thrust on them. In such a situation the mother often tends to overlook/ignore even when they see their children getting into this habit. She thinks that the child is keeping himself busy in this activity while she can finish all her work during that time. She thinks that if she makes an attempt to remove the thumb every now and then, the child would end up crying, which would again consume a lot of her time and hamper her work.

- **Absence of the feeling of emotional security**

Children tend to form the habit of thumb sucking in the absence/lack of emotional security. For example, if the mother has been unable to breast-feed her child because of certain medical problems or for other reasons, then the child starts feeling emotionally insecure and starts thumb sucking.

Sonia was an aspiring model. She continued modelling even after marriage, but had to discontinue it when she got pregnant. She was highly ambitious so she did not breast-feed her child for fear of spoiling her figure. The child started thumb sucking and continued even much after he grew up.

- **The use of soothers**

Some mothers habituate their children to soothers or use feeder (bottle) to give milk. When the children are weaned from the soother or feeder, they start sucking their thumbs.

In the opinion of psychologists sucking a soother is similar to thumb sucking. The only difference being that a soother is soft and flexible while the thumb is hard. Hence, sucking the soother is likely to be less harmful as compared to thumb sucking. Even then the use of soother is best avoided.

- **Oversight on the part of parents or relatives**

Normally all children attempt to start thumb sucking between 3-4 months of age. If it is ignored at this time then thumb sucking can form into a permanent habit. Thus the mother or grandparents should remove the thumb whenever the child tries to put in his mouth.

Some mothers feel delighted on seeing the child sucking his thumb, as they find it to be a lovable sight. They do nothing to divert this activity and the child makes it a permanent habit, which continues even as the child grows up. In addition to this, in case of working mothers the child is often in the care of grandparents or other relatives. Sometimes these people initiate thumb sucking in the child themselves thinking that the child would pacify himself thus. Repetition of the same action time and again establishes this habit permanently.

- **The feeling of hunger getting subdued**

The child sucks his thumb when he is feeling hungry, then he gets the feeling of hunger being subdued or even satiated completely. Psychologists feel that as thumb sucking makes the child feel satiated, he begins to enjoy the action.

World famous psychologist Sigmund Freud has written that in the first three years of the child, his urges and power are limited to mouth, lips, teeth and tongue.

- **Monotonous environment**

If the environment around a child remains monotonous for a long time with no positive change to engage the attention of the child, then the child in some cases starts sucking his thumb to come out his boredom. According to the World Health Organisation, the habit of thumb sucking in children depends on two main things – low level of understanding and monotonous environment.

HOW TO GET RID OF THUMB-SUCKING PROBLEM?

During the initial stages of thumb sucking it appears to be a very desirable right, but as the child forms it as a permanent habit and doesn't let go of it even as he advances in age, it assumes the proportions of a serious problem. All the efforts of the parents to make the child surrender this habit go astray as the child remains adamant about not giving up the thumb. He rather prefers to go without meals to leaving his thumb.

In normal circumstances one should not adopt strict measures to make the child give up his habit, until the habit has already had a serious impact on the child such as disfiguration of teeth, mouth and other physical problems discussed earlier. According to child specialist Dr. Freeman and child physician Dr. Alexander Lung of Calgary University, Canada, no efforts should be made to address this problem till the child himself wants to give it up.

If the child continues to suck his thumb even after six years of age, then a child physician should definitely be consulted. On your end you can take care of the following facts to make the child give up his thumb sucking habit:

- Make an effort to find out the reason behind the development of this habit. In case the child has taken up thumb sucking to alleviate his hunger or thirst, try to give him food, beverages at the right times at proper intervals.

- Do not scold the child or punish him severely for thumb sucking.
- Never criticise or ridicule the child in front of others. Such actions will only make the child more adamant.
- Do not tease the child yourself nor let him be a victim of others' ridicule. Teasing the child can aggravate the problem.
- If a fairly grown up child is continuing to suck his thumb, then he should be explained the harmful consequences of the habit and persuaded to give up the habit himself.
- If the child is suffering from an inferiority complex about something, then this problem should be addressed first.
- The child can be motivated to give up thumb sucking by giving him small incentives. Dr. Michael Lee Bovilz of Nebraska Medical Centre has listed quite a few measures in his research to cure the child of this habit. He has said that the child should definitely be rewarded if he has not put his thumb in his mouth for a whole day. Dr. Michael found out in the course of his research that 12 out of 22 children stopped thumb sucking in a period of 3 months, when given small incentives. After that during his study in a year he found out that around 85% gave up their habit.
- If the child has a habit of sucking his thumb in his sleep, then slowly remove the thumb from his mouth. Give a small toy in his hand instead.
- According to Dr. Freeman, the biggest treatment for this problem that can be given, is not ignoring or dismissing this habit. This problem is more self-centred in nature.
- Do not intervene in his habit too much. Children tend to

get more attracted towards forbidden activities. It is the normal tendency of a child to do just the opposite of what he is asked to do.

- You can coat the thumb and nails of the child with a harmless bitter paste available with the chemists for this very purpose. The paste can be applied during night or during the time when the child tends to suck his thumb the most. It is also advisable to tell the child before applying the paste.
- Always tell the child before hand if you feel it necessary to wrap his thumb with a Band-Aid, gauze etc. to dissuade him from sucking his thumb.
- If the child still is unable to get over his habit by any of these measure, then consult a child specialist for the problem. Specialists can put such instruments in the child's mouth which will make it impossible for him to suck his thumb.

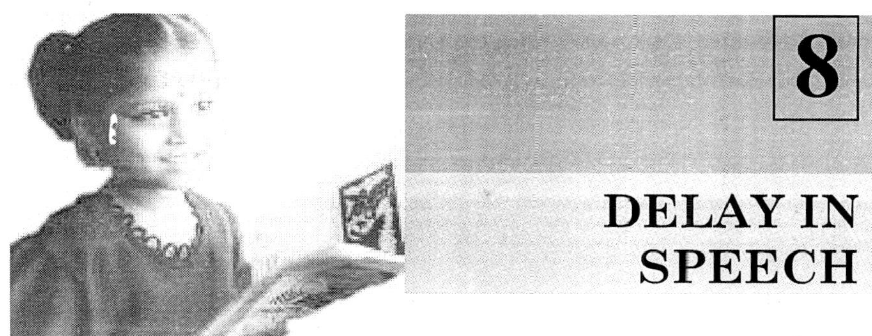

8

DELAY IN SPEECH

Rita's two year old daughter Jyoti was becoming a major cause of worry for her. Despite being two years of age, her daughter could not speak beyond "mamma", "papa" and other such simple words. Rita's growing concern found her speaking about her daughter's problem before anyone who came to their house. Rita's mother-in-law dismissed Rita's fears as baseless as she thought that it is normal for some children to start talking a little late. This did not convince Rita as she would see her brother's son, aged one and a half years speak much more than her daughter. Jyoti had begun sitting and walking at the right time, only her speech was delayed.

On the other hand even though Sudha's two and a half year old daughter Payal faced a similar problems as Jyoti, Sudha was totally unconcerned. Sudha's elder son too had started talking a little later; therefore, Sudha assumed that Payal too would be no different from him. Payal communicated with Sudha and all others with the help of symbols.

Sudha's friend Pushpa came to visit her with her six year old son Sonu. Sudha was surprised to see that Sonu could not speak clearly at all and that his speech could not be understood at all. Pushpa explained that when Sonu had started speaking she had not paid much attention to his speech. As she could understand most of the words Sonu uttered, she thought that others would begin to understand as well. But his speech never improved much. Pushpa remarked that though Sonu is much better than before, it will take some more time before he can speak normally.

On seeing Payal, Pushpa advised Sudha to consult a speech therapist at this stage itself so that any particular problem can be corrected at this very stage and before it develops into a bigger problem.

Children often suffer from many speech related problems such as delay in speech, inability to speak or unclear speech or lisp in speech. Whatever the problem, parents should pay immediate attention to it.

Some parents remain casual towards such problems, while some others panic so much that they keep running from one physician to the other out of the fear that their child might never be able to speak in the future.

If the child is suffering from any of the above problems and is over two and a half years of age, parents should consult an E.N.T. (Ear, Nose, and Throat) specialist. Apart from this it is advisable to consult a speech therapist as well.

POSSIBLE CAUSES

Most of the speech related problems of children such as delay in speech, absence of clarity in speech etc. may have physical or behavioural causes behind them. Behavioral causes/ problems can be easily addressed. The main causes are:

- **Understanding the child's non-verbal/symbolic communication**

When some children turn one-two years of age, they start communicating with signs instead of attempting to speak. They have their own symbols and signs for basic requirements like water, toilet etc. The mother begins to comprehend the signs of the child and is naturally delighted at her little one's ability to communicate. It has to be noted here that such children never make an attempt to talk as they feel that their mother understands all their signs. But as they grow up, their hesitance to speak begins to create problems.

- **Limited knowledge of words in children**

Some children have less capacity to group words as compared to other children. Therefore, when a visitor or relatives asks them something which they are unable to understand, they respond with signs. Such children do not even try to speak the difficult words. They use minimum words to communicate and just about manage to communicate.

But as the child nears the school going age of 3-4 years, his inability to express and understand words becomes a major concern for the parents.

- **Overwhelming love and Pampering**

Rinki was the darling of the house. She was a talkative child from the age of 2-3 years. Being extremely talkative and imaginative, she used to weave her own stories and tell them with attitude. In the process of narration she used to tongue twist words or half-pronounce them. Whenever she said "tater" for "water" or "tat-you" for thank-you", she won great applause and cheer from everyone. But slowly this turned into a habit. Even when she grew up she could not pronounce many words clearly.

Thus appreciating everything (even wrong and unmeaning

actions) that the child does and pampering him/her excessively can also spoil the speech.

- **Lack of inspiration**

The reason why some children do not speak clearly or speak late can be that the parents are too busy to pay attention to the child's speech. A child aged 2-2½ years speaks slowly and in pauses. In this stage parents have to invest more time to listen to the child completely. If parents and other elders listen attentively to the child and inspire him to express himself, he definitely picks up speech or else, if he has no opportunity to speak he begins to speak less or not speak at all.

- **Less Memory**

Some children can pick up and retain smaller words and phrases, while they find it difficult to pick up and retain long or difficult words. Some children do not have a strong memory and they find it difficult to memorise the syllables and sound of the word in the correct sequence. Such children speak less, speak late or speak unclearly in nervousness. However, this problem can be eliminated with proper practice.

- **Overburdening the child beyond his capacity**

Some highly ambitious parents want to make their child intelligent and smart from his initial years itself so that he is widely appreciated. Let us see Vipul's case now, who was born of a Bengali mother and a Punjabi father. Both parents aspired that Vipul should learn their respective languages. Similarity both grandparents too tried their hand with teaching Vipul their styles. At school Vipul was exposed to English and Hindi. Now the child got completely lost in the mire of so many languages and started mixing words from these languages. This confusion gradually took its toll on Vipul and he started speaking a blurred manner.

In addition to parents, it is also the duty of the teachers to see that they are not overburdening the child beyond his age capacity.

- **Pessimistic attitude/intolerance of the parents**

Children love to make noise and create complete ruckus when they play. Some parents or grandparents are intolerant towards this noise and often take the children to task stringently. Too much disciplining/punishments etc. scare the children who then prefer to keep mum to avoid such measures.

- **Fears**

Some children are highly sensitive. If they are scolded or beaten, they become terrified and nervous out of fear and either refrains from opening their mouth in front of strangers or start speaking minimally.

PHYSICAL CAUSES

Some children face problems in their speech because of certain physical problems. Such problems need to be addressed also by a speech therapist, along with individual behavioural changes on the part of parents, teachers etc. A speech therapist can help cure the physical problems to a great extent.

- **Low Intelligence Quotient (I.Q.) of the child**

Some children have relatively low I.Q. from their birth. They are unable to learn or grasp new words easily. Therefore, they are unable to speak clearly for a long time.

- **Weak audibility**

Audibility (the capacity to hear/listen) has a very important role in development of speech. Any child or adult first has to hear the word being pronounced to grasp it and to record it in his memory. Vocabulary of a child is developed only because of hearing new words. If the child has weak audibility, his speech too suffers consequentially as he hasn't heard enough words to produce it on his own. In this situation he will either speak in an incorrect way or speak much later.

- **Long illness etc.**

If the child has suffered from a fairly long spell of illness/fever during his initial years, his speech is likely to get affected. The child develops his vocal chords etc. by one year of age and is ready for speech then. If due to any reason he is ill for a prolonged period at his time, then it can cause a delay in his speech as well.

- **Any form of damage to the brain**

In a high degree fever or any injury, if the brain has suffered an injury as well, then the child loses his ability to comprehend the meanings of words. It becomes a mammoth task for such a child to develop his language/mental vocabulary. At times if the child has a congenital brain defect at the time of birth, he may not able to speak at all.

During pregnancy if the mother has suffered from a long illness, and the brain of the fetus has been affected, the child may not be able to speak clearly when he grows.

- **Other physical deficiencies/problems**

If there is an anomaly in the tongue or lips of the child, he loses his ability to speak properly or he may become mute for life. All these organs of the body are speech related organs. All these organs have to be completely developed and healthy for the child to speak to be able to normally.

Suggestions to Control the Problem

Normally toddlers of 8-9 months start mouthing monosyllabic sounds like 'ma, pa, bua', etc. and some other children start speaking single words at 10-11 months. By the time the child is 1½-2 years of age, he is able to speak half a sentence or even a complete sentence. If at this age, any child doesn't speak at all, then it is advisable to see a doctor immediately and consult a speech therapist.

Doctors and speech therapists conduct an audiometric test (audibility test) of the child to find out if the child is suffering from any problem associated with hearing. Apart from this the general aptitude of the child is also tested by means of various games.

If the child speaks less, unclearly or lisps while speaking, then parents should meet a speech therapist without fail. Speech therapists can bring about a great improvement in the child's speech by practicing and with the help of various special techniques.

Even parents should pay attention to the following things and try to bring about an improvement in the child's speech:

- Do not encourage the sign language used by small children. Bring him to speak rather than explain with signs.
- Even parents should avoid speaking with symbols in front of the child. For example, if you begin to close your eyes etc. and use it as symbol for sleeping, he too will start making use of signs to communicate as he would find it easier than speaking.
- Make it explicitly clear to the child that if he wishes to get any of his wishes fulfilled, he will have to communicate it verbally. Simultaneously also provide him adequate time to speak his mind.

- Encourage the child to speak. Listen to him patiently and talk to him as well. Give the child an opportunity to speak to guests, relatives etc. when they pay a visit.
- Whenever the child misspells any word, or pronounces it wrong, explain the correct way of pronunciation to him. Do not interrupt or taunt him in front of guests/relatives. Teach him right speech when he is with you alone.
- It is pretty natural for you to love your child's lisped speech (Totli boli). But it is not right to talk with her/him in the same manner. If you also talk to him in lisped speech, then the child will not be able to learn the right manner of speaking. Lisping is the natural early speech of the child. But your repetition of the same will reinforce this very speech as the correct form of speaking. Whenever the child lisps, you should in fact repeat the same set of words in the correct form.
- Similarly the class in charge/class teacher should also correct the child's lisped speech by showing him the correct pronunciation. The teacher should give every child an opportunity to speak and express himself. Particular attention should be given to children who speak less/ speak unclearly.
- Give your child an opportunity to play and mix up with other children. This increases the word power and language of the child. It is easier for the child to pick up words spoken by his peer group. Playing with other children also increases the practical knowledge of the child.
- Never pressurise your child to speak. Also never scold, taunt or make fun of him if he refuses to speak with guests/ relatives etc.
- If your child is speaking in front of guests, never cut him

short or scold him in between. Encourage your child to speaks.

- As the child begins his initial speech, familiarise him with the names of everyday things by repetition and regular use of such words. This way he will effortlessly learn the name of the things, which will increase his vocabulary as well.
- Do not jump into completing the child's incomplete sentences. Give him time and let him complete them himself. In your spare time teach him phrases and small sentences.
- Encourage the child to speak using the medium of story telling, poems, toys etc. When the child recites a poem or a story, give him his due appreciation and applause.
- Play games which give the child an opportunity to speak.
- Do not enjoy or appreciate the child's attempts to pronounce the words in the other way around, lisped speech and wrong imitation of other people. If you do not correct the child, he will think his wrong speech to be right. Then he will adopt that very mannerism of speaking in the future as well.

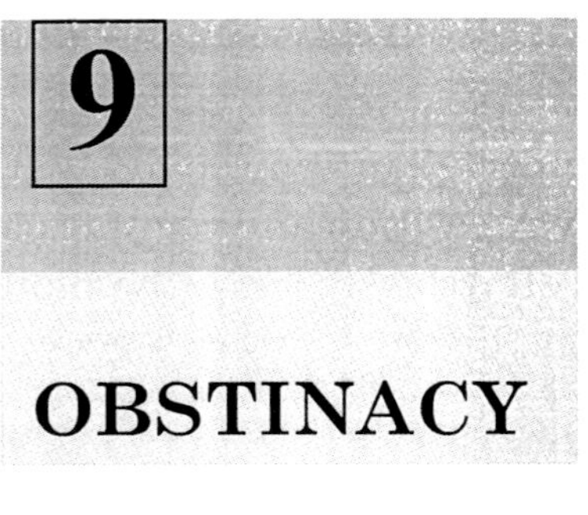

9 OBSTINACY

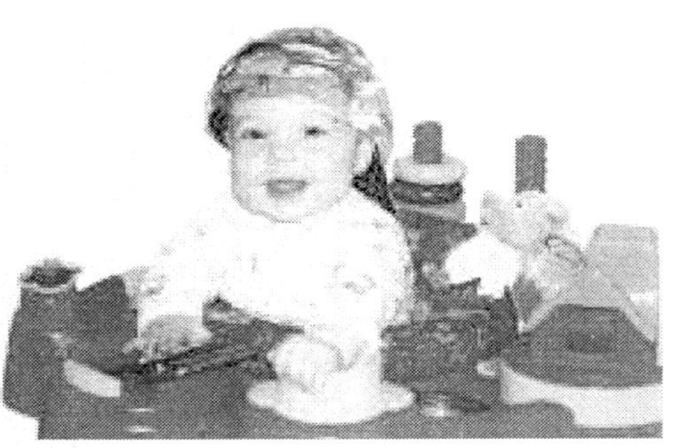

Obstinacy is a very common problem in children. In all the families, we would find children who obstinate for one thing or the other. Main reason for children's such behaviour, it may be said, is that nuclear families are developing. Every such family has one or two children, even if they are not able to run their own expenses well. This way, children are used to such atmosphere that they don't want to listen 'No' and they obstinate for every denial.

Let us try and understand obstinacy through these two case studies.

"Kshitij is an extremely undisciplined and obstinate child. His rude and foul answers or responses always shock his parents and family members. His behaviour becomes even worse when they have guests over. His parents are unable to find out the cause of his rebellious and undisciplined behaviour."

"Shilpi displays extreme sets of behaviour at different occasions which leaves her mother aghast. At times she is an extremely obedient and industrious child, completing her homework on time and coming first in her class: At other times, if her wishes are not adhered to, she starts shouting and crying in the middle of the road or a shop if her parents do not buy her the article she desires at that time."

These are common problems that contemporary parents face. On their end, they try to bring about change in the child's behaviour by making them understand and when the children refuse to listen to them, parents forcibly resort to harsh methods like admonishing or physical punishments (beating etc.). However, the latter methods leave both the parents and children troubled and offer no solution in the real sense. Similar is the case with Mrs. Meera Sharma and her son John. John has a very short-tempered and an impatient nature. Whenever things do not go his way, he starts hitting his head against the wall to show his anger and displeasure. Mrs. Sharma is completely clueless as to how her five year old has acquired this habit and about what is it that she can do to change this.

In order to solve problems pertaining to children, we must pay attention to their root cause. But even before that, it is important that we understand certain things related to child behaviour.

Every child is complete and unique in his own way. Some of his habits and actions may be similar to other children and some may be different altogether. Therefore, two children should never be compared to each other and should never be expected to behave in the same way. Even in the same situations children have different habits and difficulties at different ages. Thus it is important to pay attention to their age before expecting a certain "appropriate behaviour" from them. From lying to stealing to obstinacy, almost every problem associated with children has a psychological reason behind it.

POSSIBLE CAUSES OF OBSTINACY

The source of most of problems of children can be traced to

their homes. Child psychologist, Dr. Bhalla believes that, "The atmosphere at home always plays a very crucial role in the development and personality of the child."

- **An attitude of indifference or neglect towards the child**

If the child has not been getting adequate love and attention of his parents, he is bound to acquire an inferiority complex due to the feeling of neglect.

If the parents are not paying enough attention to child because they are pursuing extremely busy careers, or have a hectic social life or the child has been left for long hours in the custody of the maid or governess, etc; the child starts feeling "unloved" or neglected. This feeling manifests itself by way of the child becoming obstinate or rebellious.

- **Tension at home**

A tensed atmosphere at house can also be equally dangerous for children. According to the child psychologist, Dr. Vineeta Paul, "If there is always a struggle and discord between parents, the home has a very chaotic atmosphere and there is an absence of harmony. In such a condition, children become uncontrollable and obstinate. As they witness a disturbed atmosphere at home, right from their childhood, they start believing that this kind of atmosphere prevails everywhere else too. They start becoming glum: "They get irritated at every other thing and also become obstinate."

Child specialist Mrs. Gita Kapoor is of the opinion that children do not have a sense or knowledge of right and wrong when they see their parents fight. Sometimes they believe their mother to be right, thereby becoming bitter towards their father and at other times, they become bitter towards their mother, believing their father to be right. In this process, the feeling of bitterness always remains in them and they end up being rebellious and short tempered as they grow.

There is one more aspect in this situation. In order to win over children to their respective sides, parents often give different temptations to lure children, even fulfilling their undeserved desires at times. The children take complete advantage of the situation and fulfil all their wishes at that time, which parents wouldn't agree to at other times. In the process, however, obstinacy and arrogance become a part of his character.

- **The parent's incapability to be determined in their 'No'**

The child's obstinate behaviour and making a show of themselves before others can be a source of embarrassment for the parents. Sometimes the parent's incapability to stick to their 'No' can also encourage children to be obstinate. Let us see a small instance to understand the concept better. For instance, if you have forbidden your child to play near the road for fear of traffic etc. and your child goes on persisting that he will play now nowhere but that particular place. When he starts throwing tantrums, you finally agree in exasperation unable to argue with him anymore. Now this may appear to be tension relieving for the moment, but it sends very wrong messages to your child. He will take it for granted that every time he persists on a thing already forbidden by you, you will finally give up if he continues with his dramatics. This may also be the case when he is insisting on watching a TV programme that you don't allow him to. Suppose guests arrive at that time and he continues with his pestering, and you let him watch TV so that you can give time to your guests, the child will understand that you are vulnerable before guests and he can exploit you then.

Many times parents, who are unstable in their decisions, are unable to decide what is good and bad for their children in the long run. Such parents prohibit the child from doing something one day and the next day or sometime later they themselves ignore the same. This action creates confusion in the young mind as well between right and wrong, acceptable and unacceptable behaviour. Such children just want to fulfil their demands by creating a scene before others, crying etc.

SUGGESTED MEASURES TO ADDRESS THE PROBLEM

As also emphasised earlier, it is the duty of both the parents to build and maintain a congenial and loving atmosphere at home. They should devote time towards their children and try to discuss their actions and pay attention to what they say. The most important thing in this regard is that parents should be stable in their decisions and stick to their "No" once they have said so. Parents should never be wavering in any situation.

If you feel that the demand of the child somewhat reasonable and feel that the child will ultimately have his way, agree to his demand in the first go itself. Never give him an opportunity to think that his tantrums can manipulate your decisions.

In the best interest of the child, both parents should consult amongst themselves first before coming to any conclusion: It is important for both parents to agree first, One's "Yes" and the other's "No" to the same situation can result in an indecisive, unstable condition. Apart from this, whatever the circumstance, one must never fulfil unreasonable demands of children, nor should one attempt to fulfil each and every demand put forth by the child.

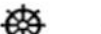

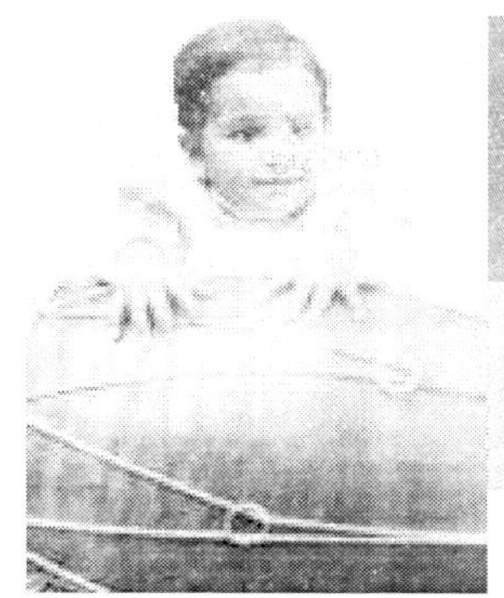

10 YOUNGER CHILD MORE OBSTINATE, WHY?

Ritik was the only son of the well-to-do Sharma family. Being the first child, he was the apple of the eye for the whole family. Parents, grandparents, uncle, aunt... no one let him be alone for even a second. All his cries were attended to promptly by one or the other the family members. Amidst all the love and pamper, Ritik soon turned four. His parents started sending him to school. Soon, Ritik found his parents and grandparents asking him if he wished for a younger brother or a sister, who could play with him and give him company. Ritik naturally was happy at the thought of a young one's entry in the family. After a while Ritik had a young brother, who was christened Sujal. Ritik's happiness knew no bounds. He played with Sujal, but whenever he expressed a desire to hold him, no one would let him for fear that he might drop the baby by mistake. This was something that Ritik detested.

Time flew by and the young Sujal turned one and a half years. Now Ritik was reprimanded by his parents and grandparents every now and then. If by chance, Ritik picked up Sujal and he started to cry, Ritik would be blamed for being mischievous with the baby and making him cry. As Sujal grew older, he turned into an obstinate child. All his demands were met on the pretext that he was younger of the two kids. However, on the other hand Ritik's demands were termed in unreasonable and he was expected to behave in a more mature way, being the elder one. It so happened many a times that for a mischief done by the Sujal, Ritik was taken to task. His parents scolded him saying that being the elder one, he did not even try to stop Sujal.

It is not uncommon that in most households after the birth of the younger child, (whether boy or girl) he/she becomes the centre of attraction for everyone at home. Whatever he does is a source of great delight for everyone. It was a similar situation when the elder child was at that stage. Even his mischiefs were enjoyed. But now that with the passage of time, he was grown a little older, he is expected to behave in a mature and responsible way being the "elder" of the two children. At the same time, the younger one is still too "small" to be scolded etc.

Now the younger one too inadvertently understands this pampering. Even though he is still incapable of understanding most things, yet, he completely understands that his demands and wishes are fulfilled and many times his elder brother or sister is scolded or beaten because of him. Gradually his tantrums increase. By the time he is 10-12 years old, he becomes so obstinate and adamant that it becomes very difficult for the parents to control him.

As an instance, let me cite an incident. Once, while returning from a trip to Shimla, once I got an opportunity to travel in a fairly crowded train. In this jostle, one family attracted my attention. The train was jam packed and this couple was travelling with two kids aged about 9 years and 4 years. There was only seat by the window, where they had seated their 4 years old, who was completely enjoying the trip with her snacks. After a while, the elder one, who was sitting on the opposite berth all this while, expressed a desire to sit by the window. At this her parents blurted out, "Can't you sit quietly? Don't you see there is such a shortage of space?"

Once the elder girl asked for water and she was handed less than half a glass and was told not to ask for it again as the journey was a long one and the water was less. In less than a minute, the younger one too demanded water as the chips she had been nibbling all the time which were very spicy. She consumed close to two glasses of water. When the elder one asked for more and began to draw a comparison, her mother made her quiet saying that her sister was too young to understand and that she being the older one should behave in responsible manner.

I would like to share one more instance which happened to me recently. I was on a trip to Europe. Many Indian families were travelling with us. One family had an elder daughter who was class Xth student (about 15 year old) and the younger daughter was about seven or eight year old. Although seven year old child is much mature and able to understand the situation, but that girl always quarrelled with other children for space in bus or food or ice cream or something else. She wouldn't own wear her shoes in the bus. She was so obstinate that she would start crying with lot of tears, if her wish was not fulfilled by her parents. I was surprised to see her behaviour. At same time, her mother clarified the situation which was really funny that how parents get befooled by their child's tantrums. She said that the younger daughter was very-very dear to them and to the whole family as she was born after a long gap. She had two-three abortions before her. So everybody loved her very much and every of her demand has to be fulfilled to keep her happy. So you can see how the younger child became more obstinate.

I hope you will agree with me that such discrimination and so much pampering will definitely make the younger child more obstinate. If parents go on fulfilling each and every demand of the child, it can also have various other negative consequences, such as:

- The two children start viewing each other more as opponents rather than as companions. This way jealousy and hatred replaces feelings of love and affection.
- The elder child develops an inferiority complex. He feels neglected and starts thinking that his parents love the younger child more.
- Even after growing up, the children are unable to resolve their differences and it may so happen that they start fighting over the parent's property on a later stage.

Thus, in most cases the responsibility of making the younger child obstinate rests with none other than parents. It is important therefore that you adopt an almost similar behaviour with both and avoid any kind of discrimination. If you scold the older child, when they quarrel, you should make sure that the younger one too is reprimanded for his mistake. It is but natural to expect the elder child to be more "responsible". But it is better and also in his interest to make him understand the situation calmly at leisure, rather than scold him when the two are in a quarrel. All obvious comparisons with the younger one should be clearly avoided. Obstinacy is a quality that should never be encouraged directly or indirectly either in the older or younger one as it will pose greater problems in the future for parents and teachers alike.

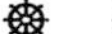

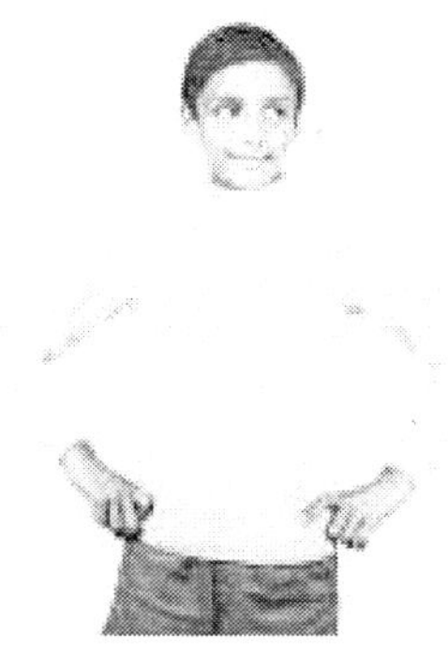

11
INFERIORITY COMPLEX IN CHILDREN

Every successful person becomes confident in his behaviour and every confident person gets success. But if the person has inferiority or superiority complex, he will never be successful. A superiority complex person might boast of his success unreasonably, but the fact is that no such complex is favourable for anybody's success. Inferiority complex in children stops his growth, development, good results in class. A child may spoil his normal behaviour on account of inferiority complex. Such child might shy, obstinate, stammering or might be facing some other problem. Inferiority complex is a root-cause of many psychological problems in children.

Sunny, a ten year old, would never join other children when they played. Instead, he would stand aloof, watching other children play in the park. He would refuse to join the children when they called him and wouldn't go even if they insisted.

One day as Sunny was standing in a corner of the park; a ball came and hit him. It injured his head and the children who were present took him home. When his mother started enquiring from "his friends", she was surprised to know that though Sunny went to the park every day, he never played with other children and never made friends there. The slightly perturbed mother asked Sunny if he had a problem with any of the children, Sunny told her sternly that he didn't like playing with other children and just wanted to be by himself. Sunny's mother Urvashi did not push him any further on this issue, but resolved to get to the root of the matter. After observing him for days, she was shocked to know that Sunny avoided making contacts with other children of his age because of the slight stammer in his speech. In other words, he was suffering from an inferiority complex because of his stammer.

Urvashi decided to act before it was too late. Gradually she managed to convince Sunny and they visited a child specialist, who asked them to consult a speech therapist for best results. Urvashi too, on her part began motivating and encouraging him to overcome his inferiority complex. Her efforts bore fruit when he started making friends and playing with them as a normal child. His sessions with the therapist removed his stammer as well and he was restored to the world of healthy and happy childhood.

Another Instance: Akash's parents changed the school he had been going to till class 6 and got him admission in a new school with better facilities. While he had always been among the top three in his class in his previous school, he was barely managing to get through in the new school. He had been promoted on 'grace' in class 7 exams and was not fairing very well in class 8 also.

His class teacher wrote to his parents expressing her concern over his performance in class. His parents consulted a child psychologist, who in the course of his sessions with Akash found that in this school, Akash had generally not been accepted by his classmates because of his dark complexion. Before he could impress his new schoolmates with his skills, he himself has become a victim of inferiority complex. His classmates had started addressing him as 'Blackie' from day one itself. His parents and psychologist made him understand that outer physical beauty is superficial. Outer beauty is not all that is there to a person. Inner qualities such as knowledge, intelligence and many other qualities are far more important than mere outer appearance. Akash gradually began to overcome his inferiority complex and started doing well academically.

Within a few years, he became the most popular among his teachers and classmates alike.

REASONS FOR INFERIORITY COMPLEX

Thus in normal course of life children become victims of such inferiority complexes due to one or the other reason. In simple words, 'inferiority complex means considering oneself inferior or lower in comparison to others'. The child starts feeling that he is useless, dull, and ugly and other such negative things. This feeling shunts his mental growth completely and doesn't let his talents blossom.

1. Inferiority complex can arise from any physical anomaly in the child (disability or handicap), being very underweight, overweight or dark-complexioned, due to a slur or it stammer in his speech, being very short-heighted, having a long or short nose or any other behavioural habit which can be made an object of humour.

2. According to child specialist, Mrs. Neena Puri, a tensed atmosphere at home or frequent quarrels between parents result in the child feeling insecure. An insecure child is unable to come out of his shell. He avoids interacting with other children as he feels that they might question him about his parents' quarrels and this way he becomes a victim

of inferiority complex. There can be many other reasons behind this too.

3. In the opinion of Dr. A.K. Sethi, "If time and again parents tell the child that he is dumb or stupid, the child actually starts believing the same. Thus one should avoid saying negative statements to the child – such as – "you are not capable of doing this," "you are too young for this," "you keep a long face always," or "you have completely spoilt your face" etc. These things kill the self-confidence in the child and give rise to inferiority complex in him which then manifests itself in many other ways.
4. Also, if parents ridicule or discuss their child's habit in detail before guests/relatives it hurts the child's self-respect. For instance, if a parent says, "Urvashi is so shy that she never greets anyone who comes to our place," time and again before other people, then he/she is are reinforcing this habit of their child. The child will be hurt and will never have the courage to greet people again in future as well.
5. Sibling comparisons can also fuel inferiority complexes. If parents constantly compare one child with the other, saying that the other one is more intelligent, good looking, hard working etc., the other child starts feeling that he is incapable, a good for nothing and acquires an inferiority complex.

SUGGESTED MEASURES TO TACKLE THE PROBLEM

Child specialist, Ms. Neena Puri has the following suggestions to this problem.

- First and foremost, we should strive to rouse self-confidence in the child. Lack of self-confidence is one of the most important reasons behind inferiority complex. A self-confident child never develops an inferiority complex. It is the parents' responsibility to recognise their child's qualities and boost his self-confidence.

- If the child has any form of physical handicap (disability), then divert his mind from his inability and concentrate on his other qualities instead.
- Keep the child away from disputes and major disagreements occurring in the family. If possible never make your child the primary witness to your quarrels. Avoid shouting etc. before the child. Go to a different room if you can.
- Never discuss or reiterate the reasons behind his inferiority complex. Also, avoid expressing your extreme sympathy for his problem.
- Consult a speech therapist for wrong pronunciation, stammering or other speech related problems. Simultaneously encourage and motivate him to make friends with other children and play with them. Also make him understand his problem and ask him to try to overcome it gradually. Develop tolerance in him so that he can take criticism, ridicule from other children in his stride and not take it to his heart and develop negative feelings within himself.
- Do not compare your child time and again with his siblings or with his friends.
- Be careful about preserving your child's self-respect. Never make fun of it.

- Develop an attitude of sharing and sociability in him. If child has been pampered badly at home and is very self-centred, do not aggravate his ego or bad habits, as this can prove detrimental in future. Inculcate a healthy temperament in your child. Avoid excessive show off or exhibitionism with your child. His dresses, toys etc. should be such that they match well with that of other children and that he doesn't stand out. Teach him/her to mix up well with other children regardless of their 'status' etc. Please understand that if your child is very dear to you, there are other parents as well who think in the same way.

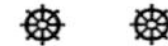

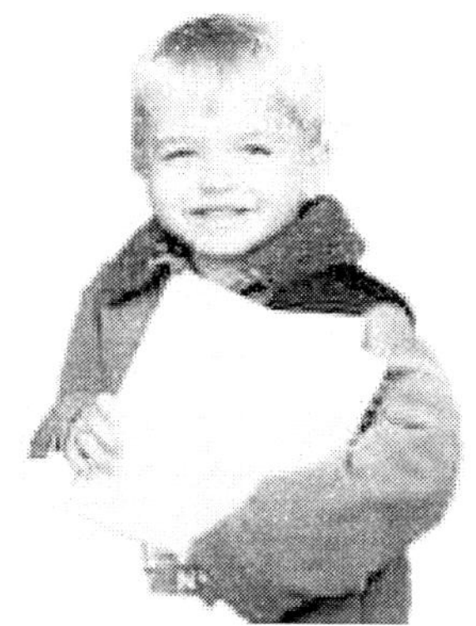

12
"PICKING UP" OR STEALING CHILDREN

Many children from the habit of picking up things from the school or from relative's bag unhesitant. In the beginning, they pick up things innocently, just to see things. They may sometime steal money from their relatives or guest's purse. But if they are not checked for their 'picking up' behaviour they get used to this habit. It is seen sometimes that some poor parents feel happy. If their child brings pencil, notebook or eraser from some other child's bag and they encourage their child to do so. It is beyond their imagination that when the child grows up, he becomes a thief or a robber. This habit of stealing should be nipped in the bud.

Anjana's mother was completely taken aback on receiving a letter from Anjana's school which read thus:

Mrs. Sharma,

"I wish to inform you that despite the fact your daughter is doing well in her studies, her habit of stealing things belonging to her classmates is becoming an issue of concern for us. She has a habit of picking up notebooks, pens, pencils and other such things belonging to other children. I have tried to make her understand through all possible means, which has been of no avail. I have tried to communicate to you many times and have sent letters through Anjana earlier too, but you have failed to respond. We wish that you please consult a psychologist about her problem. We are sorry to inform you that if we are unable to see a change in her behaviour in another 15-20 days, we will be forced to expel her from the school.

Kindly pay immediate attention to this complaint."

Anjana's mother Mrs. Sharma stood spellbound for a minute. Then she began recollecting all the incidents when she had seen new pencils, rubbers and such other things in her schoolbag and even questioned her about them. Anjana had always said that they had been given to her by her classmates on their birthdays or had been given to her as gift; Mrs. Sharma began to wonder what had given rise to this habit in Anjana. They were fairly well to do and there was never dearth of anything in the house that a child would require. Even then her daughter had started stealing things which belonged to other children. With an apprehensive mind she showed the same letter to her husband Mr. Sharma, when he returned from work that evening. Both of them discussed the situation and decided that they would take the help of a psychologist, who could find out the cause behind this habit and help them cure Anjana of this habit.

Similar was the case of 8 year old Ankit, who belonged to an upper middle class family. Being the only child, he had his hands full of latest toys, chocolates, clothes and such other things. But he acquired the habit of stealing fancy toys and other decorative items when they visited family friends. This habit of his came to the notice of his mother, when they returned from the house of his maternal grandmother after spending a few days there during the summer break. When his mother started unpacking their luggage, she saw some pieces of silver cutlery, some toys and many such items that Ankit had picked up from his grandmother's house. What she saw, she was infuriated. But she decided to control her temper and called Ankit to her room. Then she made him sit next to her and showed him the items she had discovered in the luggage. She asked Ankit how they had come in there. Ankit said proudly with a glitter in his eyes. "Mom, my magic has got these things here. "Magic"?, his mother was trying hard to control her anger. Ankit told her that he had liked the spoons at his grandmother's place and also the toys of his cousin Aashish. So he had kept them in his bag. His mother made him understand that lifting things belonging to others without their consent is termed as theft and not magic. And she also told him that stealing was a very bad and detestable habit.

Ankit's mother was determined to make him get rid of this habit of stealing. So whenever they visited family or friends and were about to leave from there, she made it a point to check all his pockets and bag and put back the things he had picked up from there. Ankit hated it when his mother put back all things he had "stolen" and once even tried to put such things in his mother's purse to avoid being caught. But when his mother saw it on returning home, she took him to task and told him in no uncertain terms, "You can tell us if you like something or are in need of it. Your father and I will get it for you. But if we ever catch you doing this again, you will not be spared." His father's name scared him and he made an effort to control his urge and gradually was able to grow out of this habit.

As is the case of Anjana and Ankit, many children develop this habit of stealing in their growing years which can become as serious issue of concern for parents and teachers equally.

CAUSES OF THIS HABIT

Before knowing more about this habit, let us first try to understand the primary causes that should lead to the development of this habit:

- **The basic tendency to acquire and collections**

Anyone can have the habit of collecting things. This may not appear to be harmful at all. But if the tendency to accumulate thing from others grows unchecked, it can often lead to stealing things. Small children cannot normally differentiate between "theirs" and "others" things. Because of their tendency to collect things, they often pickup or hide the things they like. This action leads elders to address such children as "liar" or "thief". However, we have also to understand that whenever a child hides a thing he likes and even makes stories and excuses regarding its absence, he is not trying to be cunning. He regards all this to be merely a game. If however, this habit to collect things is given a right direction and moulded in the right way, it can well prevent the formation of the habit of stealing.

- **Inquisitiveness about things**

It is the normal tendency of a child to wish to hold or touch any new thing he sees. But as elders we often do not let a child fulfil his fancy for the fear that he might break or spoil the thing. We must understand that the desire persists in the child, and he tries to get hold of the thing when he is alone, or when no one is around. Then he hides the same thing so that no one can catch him or point a finger at him. If he is successful in this once, he makes it a habit to pick up any new thing that catches his attention such as coins, pens etc. at a given opportunity.

- **A desire to display courage**

Sometimes children succumb to peer pressure and take to stealing in order to display their courage and show they are smart in front of their friends and classmates. For instance, an argument among classmates that it is not possible to lift a pen from the teacher's table in her presence can take the form of a challenge and one of them can perform the act to show his prowess. If given many situations, the child can become used to these actions and make stealing into a habit.

- **Jealousy**

The element of jealously in student life can often work as a cause in instigating the habit of stealing. Let us see an example.

Saurav, an outstanding student, always used to top in his class. This was unpalatable to many of his classmates. Just days before the exam, one of them stole all of Saurav's notes so that his preparation would suffer. This didn't deter Saurav and he still managed to score the highest marks. Next time when Saurav reached the examination hall, he was shocked to find his entire stationary missing. Somehow he managed to find a pen to write his exam.

- **Extreme discipline**

Sometimes if parents are too strict or maintain highly disciplinary atmosphere at home, children resort to stealing. Let us suppose someone brings a delicacy home. But if child has scored fewer marks in his exams or has disappointed his parents with his behaviour somewhere and is not allowed to eat the delicacy, the child will take the refusal very badly and might take the delicacy without parents' knowledge. Such incidents leave a lasting impression in the child's psyche and he might steal the same delicacy from his friends or relatives in the future too.

- **Discrimination amongst children**

It so happens in our families that we tend to pamper the younger child more than the elder one. As if by instinct, we expect the elder one to be more responsible and 'giving' towards his younger sibling. Even if parents are not deliberate in this, it does create a feeling of jealousy in the elder child. He feels angry and irritated at sharing his parent's attention with his brother- sister. Therefore in order to vent out his feelings, the elder child often hides a toy or some other item of utility which belongs to his sibling. He feels that this would bring parents to approach him for help in searching for the lost toy and give importance to him.

- **"To show off"**

Some children steal the things belonging to others so that they can "show off" in front of their friends or classmates. They distribute these fancy "stolen" articles amongst their friends to make an impression that they are well-to-do and can afford such things. In case girls belonging to ordinary middle class families who are sharing hostel with girls belonging to rich class families, they often steal cosmetics, hair clips, jewellery etc. belonging to others to show off they are no less.

SUGGESTED MEASURES TO TACKLE THIS PROBLEM

- As parents, sometimes, we become judgemental too soon. If we see a child in possession of a thing that doesn't belong to him, instead of jumping to conclusions, it is best if we talk to him about it and try to know how and why he has acquired it. As parents, it is our responsibility to try and understand the mindset of our child.
- Over-discipline often works in a negative way. Fear of punishment often prompts children to lie. Therefore it is best to approach the child in an affectionate manner.
- In the families where there is more than one child, parents should be careful about not neglecting one child over the other one. It has to be understood that while the younger baby is not in a position to comprehend much, the elder one can and needs your affection more. Try and pay equal attention to both the children.
- In situations where you find your child in the possession of pens, pencils, rubbers, which he has picked up from someone at school, ask him how and why he has got them, without being too strict. Then ask him to take them back and return them to their owners. If you decide to keep the articles, for fear of bad publicity, beware. This would inadvertently send a signal to the child that you are encouraging his actions. He will not hesitate to repeat the same action, as he will feel that by not asking him to return

the stolen articles back; you are supporting him in an indirect way.

- It is the duty of parents to provide an atmosphere that is conducive to the child's healthy physical and mental growth. Parents should be loving and sympathetic towards the child's needs and should correct his wrong habits and behaviour in a responsible way.
- Give ample opportunities to the child to develop his natural instincts. Do not keep giving him prohibitory orders.
- If you feel that you are unable to find an appropriate solution to any problem pertaining to your child, it is in the best interest of the child for you to consult a child psychologist. These days the facility of "Special Child Guidance Clinics" for children is available in all major cities where children can be taken for a consultation. Children's behaviour can be made upright and cultured with the right atmosphere and direction.

As parents one should try to avoid the occurrence of the above mentioned incidents and according to the age, capability and receptivity of the child, one should try to make the child understand the difference between "his belongings" and "others belongings".

Has the child stolen with an intention of 'stealing'?

Sometimes it becomes a little difficult for us as parents to determine whether the child has brought the article as a prank or a game or if he has actually picked it up with the intention of stealing it. Before taking a decision on whether your child has stolen a thing you see in his possession, it would be worthwhile to consider a few points such as :

- **Age of the child :** If the child is between 2 and 4 years, he would have picked the thing after getting attracted to it or acquired it playfully.

- **Has the child been picking things for a long time now?:** If the child is between 7-8 or 10 years and above, and has been picking up or stealing things from his childhood, by now, the habit of stealing would have been reinforced in him.
- **Which are the things that he steals :** It is equally important to pay attention to the things that he gets home. Does he get stationary items, decorative items or utility items? If not any of the above, does he get toffees, chocolates and other such things? After taking notice of the kind of things he gets, give a thought to the fact whether he has not been getting these things at home or have you been disciplining him at the cost of not providing him things he desires. Has he, in general, acquired a habit of accumulating things?

It would not be in the interest of the child to label him a thief at this stage. However, it would be appropriate to deeply analyse the cause behind the child's behaviour of picking up or stealing things that do not belong to him.

- Does the child belong to a family which is financially not strong enough for the parents to able to fulfil all this necessities and desires?
- What does the child do with the things he steals? Does he hide them or does he try to use them?
- How many siblings does the child have? Who else is present in the family and what kind of relation does the child have with the other members?
- Do the parents of the child have cordial relations? What kind of a relation do the parents share with the child?
- What is the age and sex of the other children in the family?
- Are both the parents working? In such a situation, is the child alone at home with a maid/governess?
- What about the friends of the child? Are they of the same age or are they elder to him? What are their backgrounds?

- Is the atmosphere at home tense? Are there frequent fights in the house? Does the child have a peaceful atmosphere to grow and develop in a healthy way?
- Is the child paying attention to his studies? What are the other activities he is involved in apart from studies?

If the child has picked up a thing that does not belong to him and tries to hide the same when questioned, or if he tries to acquire the thing with one excuse or the other, it means that child is fully aware of the fact that he has stolen the thing. He completely understands the concept of stealing and is also conscious of the fact that he can be punished for his misdeed if the truth is revealed. In such a situation he will try to hide the 'stolen thing' in his school bag, almirah or any other place and will try to use the thing without the knowledge of others.

FOR THE TEACHERS

The complete development of any child calls for equal contribution on the part of both parents and teachers. If the child has acquired a habit of stealing money or any other article, the teacher should adopt a sympathetic approach towards the child and try to address the problem through interactions with the child. The teacher should refrain from giving him punishments before the entire class.

Apart from this, the teacher should encourage and motivate the child to participate in all extra curricular activities. If the child has a high I.Q. (Intelligence Quotient) and has adopted wrong habits like stealing all of a sudden, then the teacher should try to find out the possible reasons behind this sudden change in the child. Also it is the responsibility of the teacher to keep the parents apprised of the child's activities. If the child fails to record improvement in his behaviour despite all efforts, it is in the best interest of the child to consult a psychologist or take him to "Special Child Guidance Clinics."

❁ ❁

13

EXTREME SHYNESS AND HESITATION

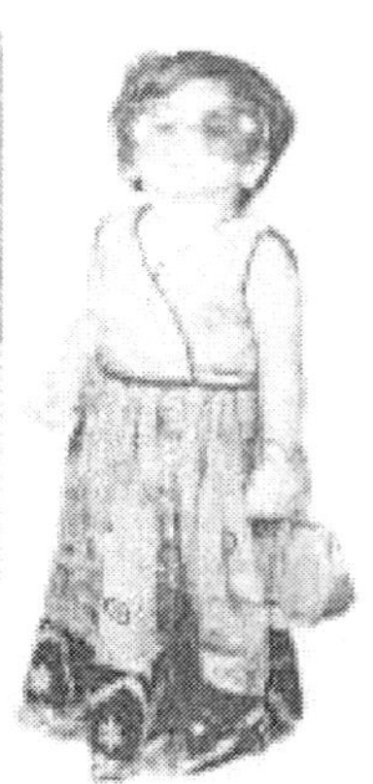

It is not uncommon to find parents complaining about the extremely shy nature of their child. Such children are quite normal before the members of their family, but turn extremely shy when guests or outsiders arrive. They try to hide behind doors and avoid saying "Hello" etc. to them.

In the initial stages parents often ignore the problem thinking that the child in general has a shy nature. But if the child continues to exhibit the same attributes even when he has turned nine-ten years of age, then the situation gets worrisome for the parents.

Some children start displaying some abnormal attributes in their behaviour when they are nervous, such as – biting their nails, sucking their thumb, stammering etc. Actually speaking, extreme shyness or excessively shy behavior is not a disease, but a behavioural problem among children.

Negative effects of excessive shyness:

- The problem of excessive shyness acts as an obstacle to the child's mental development and prevents him from developing positive qualities, such as independence and self-confidence. The lack of these qualities in turn, holds the children back from taking an active participation in group activities. Such children hesitate from participating in the co-curricular activities of the school such as sports, play acting, singing, dancing etc. on the stage in front of an audience.

- It is generally seen that shy children are unable to befriend other children in the class because of their diffident nature. If at all they attempt to make friends, they try to make friends with children who have a nature similar to theirs.
- Such children refrain from taking an active part in classroom sessions/discussions. Due to their shy nature they do not respond to the teacher's queries, despite knowing the answer and are often subjected to unnecessary punishments, ridicule etc.
- Parents of such children become extremely possessive about them and try to go out of the way to fulfil all their desires. That's when the children become used to becoming pampered and start becoming extremely dependent on others for the fulfilment of their wants. Even after they grow up and are ready to face life, they are devoid of the streak of self-reliance in their personality.
- Excessively shy children become a victim of inferiority complex. This complex prevents them from attaining a sense of self-satisfaction and they are unable to satisfy their urge of self-expression and self-respect.
- Such children are unable to come to terms with reality when they grow up. They are unable to perform well at job interviews because of their nervousness.

POSSIBLE CAUSES

Most of the behavioural problems in children stem from

personal or familial reasons. Some of the reasons that attribute to excessive shy behaviour and hesitation in children are:

- **Excessive pampering and low self-confidence**

Excessive love and pampering result the spoilt children. Some parents behave in such a way that the children are given an upper hand and a say in every situation which is totally unwarranted. They fulfil each and every legitimate and illegitimate demand of their children, thus making them materialistic. Children too begin to understand and exploit this weakness of their parents and make them an instrument of fulfillment of their wishes. Even though children are an embodiment of innocence and ignorance, yet they are intelligent enough to understand that their howling and crying can make the elders of the family (parents, grand-parents etc.). Succumb to pressure and give into their demands. Naturally so, such children turn a blind eye to their faults and give utmost importance to their desires and wants only. Many times parents, because they are tired, or because they want to avoid unnecessary commotion in the house, submit to all the demands of their children. They also complete all the chores of their children well before time. Such parents feel that they are making lives of their children easier. However they fail to understand, that by doing so, actually they are helping weakening them instead of helping them. The child never learns how to do a job assigned to him on his own and fails to understand the concept of learning by making mistakes. Also he never acquires or the feeling/concept of success or failure which he would have, had he given shape to the work himself.

In the above situations the parents' over-involvement deprives the child from taking initiatives and he is unable to take decisions, make efforts or even make a choice between two given alternatives. Thus he is not able to build his self confidence which is the primary cause of excessive shyness.

According to Dr. Suman Malhotra, it is natural and right for parents to display their love and affection towards their children. But love to the extent of pampering, ignoring all his mistakes and not counselling him for right behaviour can prove to be detrimental to their future. Children become extremely obstinate and shy, particularly so in the presence of strangers.

- **Strict disciplinary atmosphere**

As explained earlier, excessive pampering does lead to the child becoming diffident and shy. At the same time on the contrary, if the child is kept in a very strict and disciplined atmosphere, even then he might end up becoming extremely shy. For instance, if the child in a state of excitement, talks a lot before guests and is reprimanded later by the parents on how he shouldn't have said such things or shouldn't have laughed so much etc., the child becomes confused at his behaviors and decides to keep aloof in the future. He is unsure about how he should behave in front of guests and the fear of rebuke or punishment from parents at a wrong action gradually makes him shy. He starts developing an inferiority complex, loses his self confidence and turns into a shy and hesitant child.

SUGGESTED MEASURES TO TACKLE THIS PROBLEM

As parents it is our duty and responsibility to strike a perfect balance in our behaviour. Thus both extreme discipline and extreme display of love, should be consciously avoided. They should try to inculcate a feeling of selflessness and sharing amongst children. The following practices can be adopted as a matter of routine in the family which can go a long way in developing self-confidence in the child and help him overcome his shyness:

- The system of family dinner can be helpful as all members sit together and discuss different things. In this discussion children also take part and become more confident.
- Reserving some time before or after dinner for "family time" wherein every member of the family discusses the events of the day, a current topic etc. can improve child's shyness.
- Asking the child in particular, to sing a song, mimic someone or express his talent in any way before the family or even before guests will be helpful.
- Paying attention to the child and letting him know that you are always there for him will make him a confident child which will reflect in his overall behaviour and attitude.

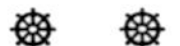

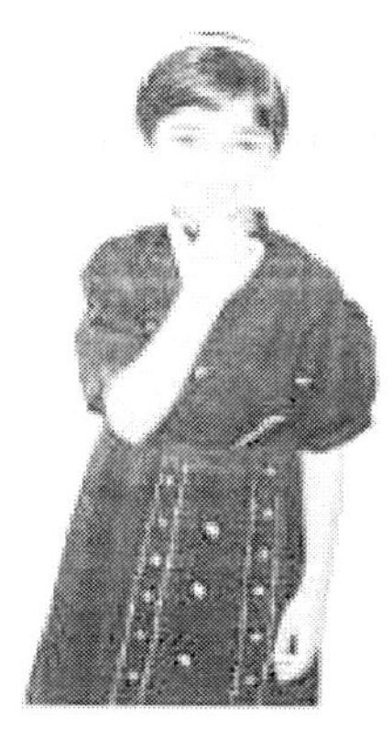

14 WHAT IF THE CHILD AVOIDS PLAYING WITH OTHER CHILDREN?

All of us are well aware of the benefits related with sports and games. It is very important for children to play. We can say it is as important as the nutritious food they eat or the love and affection they are worthy of. Games bring about the physical, mental, social and moral development in the child.

Some children like to be by themselves and play alone, while some easily mix up with other children, make friends and start playing with them. Children who prefer to be aloof are generally seen to be obstinate, irritable and egoistic. Such children want to be alone or gloomy. They keep watching other children play from a distance, but never go ahead and make friends with them. They find it difficult to play in a group.

Let me illustrate it better with Anoushka's example. Anoushka stays with her parents and grandparents and is the only child in the family. She is loved and pampered by everyone. But she prefers to play alone with her dolls and toys. She quickly hides all her toys when she is told that a child is going to come and visit them. Earlier in many instances her parents have told her to hide her expensive games and dolls as the child who is about to come to their house might break them. Now this has left such a deep impression in her mind, that Anoushka does not wish to play with any child who comes to their house, nor does she go out to play. In a family get-together or a party, three year old Anoushka just sticks to her parents and wants them to hold her, refusing to play with other children.

You will agree that Anoushka doesn't serve a healthy example. It is very important for children to play with other children. While playing, their mutual interaction with each others teaches them general behaviour, the way to present themselves before others and general knowledge in an unconscious way. As they continue conversing with each other while they play, they also develop a feeling of harmony and mutual understanding.

Under normal circumstances, children start identifying their peer from the age of 2-3 years onwards, and want to go and play with them. They also develop an instinct to make a place for themselves in a group. It is worthwhile to mention here that some children have leadership qualities from this age itself and they make other children do what they desire. They take charge and all the other children play games decided by them. On the other hand, some other children are of submissive type and they do as they are asked to. They generally follow the behavior shown by other children. Now such children shy away from groups. They feel intimidated being in a group as being of submissive nature they are unable to put their point across and are often forced to listen to others. Slowly and gradually they stop playing with other children.

It is important for your child to play with other children as this would bring about a complete development in him. If your child avoids playing in a group with other children, take a serious note of this and try to explore the reasons behind this.

POSSIBLE CAUSES

Your child may not be willing to play with other children because of the following reasons:

- **Lack of Self-Confidence**

As we have already discussed earlier, if the child has any anomaly in him such as a stammer, slurred speech, is too fat or thin, is hard of hearing, is short in height or doesn't have good features, he develops an inferiority complex about himself and loses his self-confidence. On top of that, if the child is reminded of his defects time and again by excessive pity etc. his confidence level would go on decreasing and he would start avoiding playing with other children.

- **Comparision between two children**

Lack of self-confidence can also be caused by comparison between two children. It is but natural that there are would be definite differences between two siblings. If one among them is more good looking, intelligent or in any way more talented than the other, and the parents keep drawing comparisons between the two, then the child who lacks behind in some way, starts losing his self-confidence. He then starts hesitating from mixing up with other children.

- **Justification before other**

Some parents try to justify or explain their child's weaknesses before others in this way – "Please don't take Tinku otherwise. It's just that he has not managed to gain height or that he still stammer". If your child overhears such talk, it would definitely put him down and he would hesitate from going in front of others, even if there are children with the visitors. If such incidents keep occur, then the child develops an inferiority complex, which can result in obstinacy or the tendency to be alone.

- **Physical or any other problem**

Many times other children are aware of the defect in the child and they start teasing the child. The child starts getting irritated and more conscious and from then on he avoids playing with other children.

SOLUTIONS

- **Motivation**

Even if your child is deficient in some respect, it is your duty as parents to constantly motivate and encourage him to rise above his deficiency. No child is perfect. Every child has some weakness or the other. It is normally seen that children who suffer from a physical handicap, are extremely talented in some other way. Therefore, in the interest of the child parents should try to encourage his talents rather than focusing on his weakness.

Let us suppose a child is very dark complexioned with the flat nose, but has an extremely good hand in drawing right from his childhood, then parents should focus on encouraging his drawing skills. If guests come over, they should encourage the child to show his painting/drawing etc. to them. Parents can even inform the child's teacher about the same so that the teacher too acknowledges and motivates the child to fare better in the field. When such children get appreciation, they overcome their weaknesses in due course of time.

- **Create confidence**

Try to instill confidence in the child from his childhood itself. If the child is a victim of ridicule by other children, neither discourage your child from playing with them, nor scold those children from doing the same. Instead, motivate your child to ignore them and still be friends with everyone. As your child keeps ignoring them, they too will rise above their teasing and gradually accept him as a part of their group. This type of a behaviour will not only increase his self-confidence but his tolerance too.

2. A disturbed / tensed atmosphere at home

If a disturbed/tensed atmosphere prevails at home either due to tension between parents or due to financial problems etc. then the child's mental development is hampered. The child develops an insecurity complex because of the unpleasant verbal abuses/exchanges and he starts feeling that his life is different from the lives of the other children he sees or meets.

- **Solution**

The solution to this problem lies with the parents, with the mother to be more specific. As a mother, it is important to be sensitive to your child's feelings. Do not force him to go out and play with other children if he doesn't want to.

Bunty hesitated from going out and playing with other children. His mother tired of trying to convince him to go out, then she decided to start playing with him at home. After a while she went out and asked one/two children to join them. Gradually Bunty overcame his hesitation and became friend with these children. One day when one of these children invited Bunty to his house, he went there. Initially he felt reluctant when he saw many other children there. But it was a matter of time before he made friends with all the children and started playing with them. When his mother attended the next "Parent Teacher Meeting", her happiness knew no bounds when Bunty's teacher told her that Bunty had many friends in the class now.

Correct behavioural approach of the parents alone can help the children to blossom. Even if differences do exist between the parents, they should avoid discussing differences aloud or quarrel before their children. Also, if one parent has reprimanded the child for an action of his, the other parent should not interfere and take the child's side. This type of behavior arouses confusion in the mind of the child about whether he has been right or wrong.

3. If the self-respect has been hurt

We elders give utmost importance to our self respect and

are extremely sensitive if our self-respect has been hurt by someone. Children being more emotional and sensitive are affected more adversely if their self-respect has been hurt. If someone laughs at a child over his habits or pulls his leg in public time and again, the child ceases to be normal and in due course he starts avoiding children as well as elders. He becomes withdrawn and does not wish to play with other children. Let us see Manas's case to understand the concept better.

Manas is a shy child by nature. Whenever guests come to his place, his parents want him to come and greet them. When he hesitates at first his parents start commenting on him in front of the guests, "Just see Manas. See how shy he is?" Then they start scolding him before them. "Manas, stop behaving foolishly. Come out immediately and say Hello." In case he still doesn't respond, they start criticising him openly, which becomes an object of humour for the guests. All these things hurt Manas deeply and he starts losing his self confidence with time.

- **Solution**

If a child exhibits this kind of withdrawn behaviour, instead of highlighting the behaviour, one should try and focus on other things instead. We shouldn't forget that the child's hesitation to play with other children is a problem in itself. Any ridicule, scolding or comments would aggravate the problem instead of lessening it.

We should be very tactful while dealing with such a child. If there is small child with the guests or relatives, we should tell our child to come and show his new toys or take the little guest and show him his room, toys etc. In this way our child will make friends with the new child without any pressure on him and start playing with him.

4. Selfish or self-centred nature in the child

Some children are selfish by nature from their childhood

itself. They never share or part with their belongings such as toys, chocolates, etc. but want to take such things from other children. They might even snatch things from other children. They might even snatch things they like if the owner doesn't wish to share it with him. Self-centred children want to own every item they like. Such children are so obsessive that they would break/damage things that they are denied or even go to the extent of hurting other children for the same. Other children too want to stay away from self centered children or would not include them in their play group either in school or at home. Thus these types of children often find themselves alone and stop playing with other children.

Sahil's parents are very proud of their son's domineering behaviour. They feel that since Sahil is never subdued by other children, he is a very brave child. Little Sahil took their praise to his heart and thought that he was doing a very commendable job by beating other children. His negative traits were encouraged by his parents. Gradually other children began to avoid him and stopped playing with him.

Manik's mother used to tell him that if he took his new ball outside to play, other children would snatch it from him or that he would lose it. Because of this Manik started becoming over possessive about his toys and whenever he would go out to play, he would never take his toys and only plays with toys of other children. Whenever other children would ask him to bring his toys out he would always make an excuse. Other children too stopped including him in their play and Manik was left alone. This irritated him and he developed negative habits like crying, throwing tantrums, being destructive etc.

- **Solution**

It is important that parents give the right direction to their children. They should try to make sure that they should in no way encourage the child to be self-centred. If he is self-centred by virtue of his nature, even then parents should make a conscious effort to encourage him to share his food, toys etc. with other children. However, we should bear it in mind that giving long lecturers to the child may produce no positive effect on the child. The message should be conveyed subtly to him by giving examples of day to day incidents he should be told in a non-assuming way that being in a group is fun and that sharing one's things with other children brings great joy.

In the early primary classes teachers are more exposed to such habits of children. Even teachers should spend sometime with children who are self centered and explain companionship etc. to them. During lunch break, if the children are motivated to share their food with each other, they develop traits of co-operation and affection towards each other. If teachers too have their food with the children and attend to the child affectionately, they can definitely bring about a positive change in the behaviour of the children.

When Ankita's class teacher told her mother, Mrs. Sharma about her habits in class, Mrs. Sharma was completely shocked. Ankita's class teacher told Mrs. Sharma that Ankita prefers to have her lunch alone. She scoffs at other children and doesn't let anyone sit next to her during the lunch hours. But as Ankita's class teacher began having her lunch in the class with the children, Ankita too was pulled into joining all other children.

Pushing children forcibly or scolding them to make friends with other children will not be solution to this problem. Parents and teachers have to bring about a change in the children by gradually persuading the children in their routine, day-to-day situations.

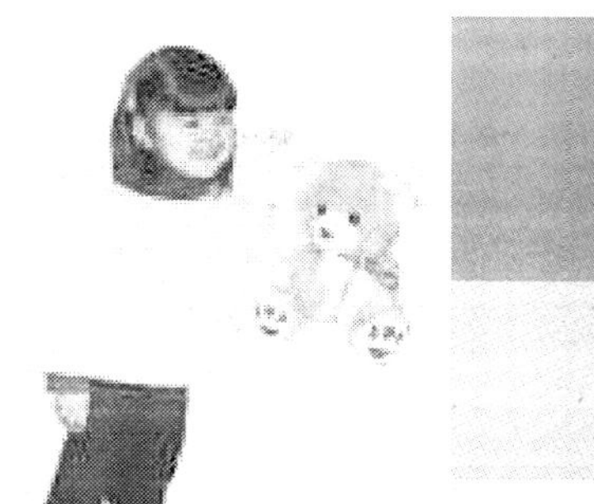

15

STAMMERING

Adults and children alike, many times are victims of the problem of stammering. In simple language a stammer can be defined as, **"speak haltingly and with unintended repetitions of sound."**

It is normal for a child aged 2-3 years to speak in a way that resembles a stammer. However at this age in life, such a speech cannot be termed as a stammer. This is the time when a child is learning pronunciation for the first time and he is experimenting and trying his hand at pronouncing various consonants. However, if the child doesn't get a conductive and healthy atmosphere at this stage, this temporarily lisps in speech can permanently change into a stammer. On the other hand, with a loving atmosphere and care by the parents, the child learns pronunciation effectively and slowly this lisp in his speech gives way to a normal speech.

According to a survey, the tendency to stammer in 1-2% children is found to be more when they are in the age of group of 2-3 years. But as I said earlier also, this can be easily overcome if the parents pay adequate attention to the child. However, if a child or an adult is a victim of this problem, and they take a strong resolve to overcome this problem, they can rectify their speech with their determination.

"Barristar Curan" is a renowned veteran in the legal arena. He swept the court rooms with his wonderful and intricately crafted arguments for hours in a row. But you will be surprised to know that Curan used to stammer in his childhood days. He was made the object of ridicule because of this habit by his friends and classmates in his school day. It so happened once that he had given his name for a debate competition at school. When his turn came and he started to speak, his speech was hindered many times because of his stammer. All through this time as he was struggling to put his views across, the other children were amusing themselves and constantly laughing.

Curan was deeply hurt because of this incident. He then took a firm resolution that he would overcome his problem and speak in such a way that no one would ever be able to utter a word while he spoke. His resolution led to him to practice his speech for long hours in closed rooms. The result was that behind these sessions of grueling practice, an orator was born, who ultimately earned great frame as an exemplary barrister after he grew up.

No doctor or specialist can ever claim that a child would stammer when he grows up, while he examines a child. This is a special type of psychological problem. Stammering is not a physical disability.

In their early years when some children speak, they get stuck in some words. At this stage some parents feel that their child is trying to speak very fast and is taking more words then he can actually speak out. They do not take note of this problem seriously. Some parents feel amused at this peculiar manner of speaking and laugh at and enjoy such speech. The child thus feels that there is nothing wrong in speaking in this way and his speech acquires a permanent stammer.

SOME FACTS PERTAINING TO STAMMERING

If your child stammers by any chance, there is no need to worry yourself that he would lag behind other children in life. Stammering is a problem that can be easily overcome by concerted efforts of teachers and parents.

If such a child is between 8-10 years of age and is mature enough, he can himself get over his problem if determines to do so in his mind. Stammering has been a subject of research in India and abroad alike. The following revelations have come out about stammering out of various studies that have been conducted so far.

- Children who stammer are completely normal in all other (mental and physical) aspects otherwise.
- It is seen that the problem of stammering starts before six years of age. Thus it is important that parents pay attention to the problem at the right time itself.
- The problem of stammering is more rampant in boys than in girls. On an average, boys are likely to be victim of this problem four times more than girls.
- Children who stammer can sing quite normally. In fact they can sing the complete song in one go without missing a beat and without getting stuck or stammering anywhere.
- It has been seen that some of the children who stammer have learnt to speak quite late.
- This problem may increase or decrease according to the situation. It will not be uniform in intensity at all times. Such children have normal speech when they are talking to children either younger to them or when they are addressing their pets. But in a classroom, when the teacher asks them to respond, the stammer may intensify. The same may be the case when these children are talking to elders

or to strangers. This problem is at its peak when these children are giving a speech etc.

- Some children who suffer from this problem may be suffering from muscular in coordination.
- It has been observed that children who stammer also acquire other behavioural problems such as nail biting, bed wetting, becoming introvert or shy, low self-confidence, throwing tantrums while eating food, thumb sucking, getting frightened easily etc.
- It has to be kept in mind that such children are highly sensitive and get baffled and lose their self-confidence very soon.

POSSIBLE CAUSES OF STAMMERING

As I also said earlier stammering is a behavioural problem and not a disease. Stammering can be a result of the following reasons:

Behavioural Reasons

• Carelessness in Speech

Suppose a child pronounces certain words in the other way and if parents consider this as a temporary lisp or they ignore the anomaly in speech, then child starts stammering gradually.

• Wrong Manner of Speaking

If on an initial level the child unknowingly or deliberately mispronounces certain syllables or words, then the attention that he gets from others often changes such speech into a stammer.

• Short Tempered or Extra Disciplinary Attitude of Elders

If parents have the habit of being very strict with the child of if they scold/terrorise the child for every small mistake, then the child becomes submissive and frightened from within and his speech starts getting slurred out of fear. Let us see an example.

Sheena was only three years elder to her younger brother. She was the centre of attraction of the family before her brother was born. She was loved and pampered a lot by the elders of the family. Things changed drastically for Sheena after the arrival of her brother. She would be scolded or taken to task for even a small mistake of hers and would be constantly taunted that being the elder one she should be more responsible now. Once it so happened that the Sheena was asked to fetch milk by her mother. Sheena was watching a cartoon at TV at that time and so got up a little late hesitantly. When her mother yelled at her for being late, the little girl dropped the glass of milk in complete terror of her mother. On hearing the loud noise and seeing the mess Sheena's mother lost her temper and gave her two slaps. On hearing the noise, Sheena's uncle who was there at that time came and shouted at her. She started to stammer while she was rendering an apology to her elders. Then she broke into tears.

Thus her mother's bad temper changed a normally speaking little girl into stammerer. After this, Sheena would always stammer whenever she was scolded or when she would be frightened. This habit continued even as she grew into a young lady.

- **By Intimating Others**

Ritwik's friend's uncle had a habit of stammering. Whenever Ritwik would return from his friend's place after playing there, he would intimate his friend's uncle in front of his mother. His mother would laugh and enjoy the act put by him. His mother would then encourage Ritwik to repeat his imitation before others as well. Little was she aware, that by doing this, she was encouraging Ritwik to spoil both his habits and his speech.

As he continued undeterred, Ritwik himself started speaking in the same way as his friend's uncle. Thus many a times imitating people who stammer can also induce this habit in children.

- **Discriminatory Attitude of the Parents**

If parents discriminate between two children in the same family i.e., if they are partial towards one child more, it can lead to the problem of stammering in the other child. If there are two or more children in the same family and the parents appear to shower more love on one child over the other, the child who feels neglected can acquire an inferiority complex and become a victim of "stammering".

- **Excessive Pampering**

If in the initial stages of the problem, the parents exhibit excessive love for the child by hugging him, kissing him etc, the child in his heart feels that the love and affection he is showered with is because of his stammering. He keeps on repeating this, so that he continues to get the attention of his parents. In this way he acquires a permanent stammer in his speech. Therefore, the parents and other elders should correct the child's speech immediately and not pity him or pamper him. It is not in the child's interest to pamper the child beyond a certain limit.

PHYSICAL REASONS

- **Any Injury at the Time of Birth**

If during the process of birth, the child suffers from an injury on his head, in particular, it can damage his nerves (ligaments). Because of this when the child grows up, he acquires this speech defect.

- **In appropriate Mental Development**

If the mind (brain) of the child has not developed according to his age or if parents try to teach him more than his mind can take at a particular age, his mental development comes to a halt. If parents pressurise on the child to learn more than his natural capacity, his mental development is hindered and his voice is disturbed, because of which the child starts to stammer.

Three year old Sharad was an extremely brilliant child. He could memorise things effortlessly. His mother made him memorise many poems one after the other, seeing the bright talent in her son. She used to ask Sharad to recite the poems in front of the guests who came to their house. Sharad too recited English and Hindi poems before them with equal ease.

This naturally impressed anyone who visited their house and people showered praises on Sharad for his talent at such a young age. Gradually his grandparents started making him learn religious hymns and songs and his uncle and aunty started making him learn other things like current affairs etc.

This created a confusion in Sharad's little mind as to what all he should memorise. In his confusion he started mixing up information that had been taught to him. In the beginning people thought that he was trying to be funny and ignored it. But as the poor child continued with his mental confusion, his parents and the other relatives started to reprimand him badly which scared him. He would now suddenly stop while reciting something. Later, this very action resulted in Sharad acquiring a stammer.

MEASURES TO OVERCOME STAMMERING

If you get the feeling of a stammer in your child's speech, even if it may be very obvious, you must immediately take notice of the same and try to keep the following things in mind. If you pay attention to this problem in its initial stages, then this is a problem that can be easily cured at home also.

- **Do not interrupt the child**

When the child is trying to express himself to you, you should pay complete attention to him and listen to all that he has to say. Do not interrupt him time and again when he speaks. When a small child begins his speech, it is normal for him to stammer/pause a bit or speak in pauses. Do not reprimand him for the same and never ask him to hurry up.

- **Do not force the child to speak perfectly**

If the child is not speaking perfectly initially, it is not proper to put pressure on him by saying such things as, "Speak properly", "Repeat this sentence", "Speak slowly", "Take a deep breath and speak again" etc. This would make the child extremely conscious and he would be scared to speak out of the fear of making a mistake. Therefore, let him first complete his sentence the way he is speaking. Advise/Correct him later in a non-formal, casual manner. If you observe that your child is facing difficulty in pronouncing a particular word, do not force him to repeat the word over and over again especially in the presence of other guests or relatives.

- **Do not ridicule the child**

If the child stammers or speaks in between pauses, parents or teachers should never ridicule this mannerism of the child. If the child is trying to say something to you and is getting stuck in between, do not hurry him up by completing phrases yourself. Give him time to think and then complete his sentence himself. Be patient and listen to him. If you create confidence in child by giving him freedom to speak, his stammering problem will soon be removed.

- **Give him to speak**

Let the child speak in his flow, at his own speed. Do not complete sentences yourself and never ask him to wrap up quickly. If you do this, this will send a message to the child that he is incapable of finding the right words and would instill an inferiority complex in the child. He would then struggle to find correct words before you do and this would only pressure on him and aggravate his stammer. Therefore, give him adequate time to speak. The best time to have a long conversation with your child is bedtime, as both you and the child are fairly relaxed at this time. This can be an ideal time to read out bedtime stories to him or to listen to his activities of his day, or about his friends, teachers etc.

- **Make him practice speech**

It is important that a stammering child practices speech. This work is best suited to the mother as a child is completely relaxed and unhesitant before his mother. Make your child face the mirror and practice his speech. If the child is hesitant initially, encourage him by saying that he looks very good while speaking in front of the mirror. This will motivate the child to practice in front of the mirror.

- **Do not make comparisons**

One should not make comparisons between the manner of speaking of any two children. Such comparisons should particularly be avoided if you are comparing a child who stammers with the one who has a normal speech. Comparisons and criticisms increase the problem instead of alleviating it.

- **Maintain a peaceful atmosphere at home**

Try and avoid quarrels and unpleasant exchanges at home. A trouble some atmosphere at home gives rise to negative feelings in the mind of the child and he acquires the habit of stammering.

Also make sure that your child has a nutritious and balanced diet. Develop a positive attitude towards life in him. Healthy and energetic body and mind are home to good habits.

- **Own a pet animal or bird**

It has been observed that children who stammer love to

talk to their pets. What is amazing is that such children do not even stammer while talking to their pets. Thus, if you have a pet at home, your child will talk to him and in the process, he will also practice his speech. This will boost the child's self-confidence and remove his stammer.

- **Pay attention to your own language and style as well**

If the members of the family, that is, grand parents, parents, elder brother/sister etc. pay equal attention to their manner of speaking and speak with decorum then the young one too will learn to speak properly. Also the child will not be affected from any type of speech difficulty.

- **Build Self-confidence**

Appreciate your child if he completes any job assigned to him. Give him his due praise. This will increase his self-confidence. Motivate him to make friends. This will give him inner strength. Make him happy and also cure his stammering.

- **Concentrate on the child's complete physical and mental development**

It is very important to keep in mind the child's age, strength and capacity before assigning any type of physical or mental (memorising extracts, poems etc.) work to him so that the child does not feel burdened or stressed. Excessive burden or stress on the child can be a cause for initiating the problem of stammering.

Also see to it that your child does not get physically over tired and protect him from diseases to the possible extent. Stammering increases during illness and weakness.

- **Give complete rest to the child**

Children who stammer need more rest as compared to normal children as stammering consumes a lot of energy of the child. Make sure that the child has a comfortable place to take rest and sleep. If possible, let him sleep in a separate room.

Children who stammer need at least ten hours of uninterrupted sleep. If it is feasible and if the child desires, let him sleep for an hour or two in the day time as well. Let him sleep as much as he wants. Do not restrain or curb his speech because of his stammer.

- **Cultivate a habit of reading aloud**

Read books and stories aloud in front of such a child and encourage him to do the same too. Reading aloud will let him overcome his hesitation and build his self-confidence. As he continues with his habit, he will even gradually forget his stammer and start speaking and reading normally.

THE ROLE OF SCHOOL AND TEACHERS

- **The school atmosphere**

The atmosphere of school should be such that the child who is a victim of this problem should not feel isolated or secluded there. Also education should be such that it is in accordance with the nature and requirement of the child.

There is absolutely no necessity for the children who stammer to be sent to special schools as stammering is neither a form of illness nor a handicap. This is a behavioural problem which can be easily cured with behavioural assistance from teachers and other students.

- **Empathetic behaviour of the teachers**

While holding a class if such a child raises his hand to answer a question, the teacher should not be impatient and give him time to answer his question. If the teacher gets impatient or scolds a child for stammering, the child will get demoralised.

If the child has been keeping quiet for a long time, the teacher should encourage him to participate in the class.

If the school has a facility of a speech therapist then the parents can seek his help.

- **Controlling and disciplining the other students of the class**

The teacher should discipline the other students of the class in such a way that they do not tease the child. The teacher should make the other students co-operate with this child and also make sure that the students do not tease the child for his stammer outside the class in the teacher's absence. If the other co-students display affection and sympathy towards the child who stammers, it will give him self confidence and help him get over his problem. On the other hand, if they tease this child or do things that make him get conscious of his weakness, it would create inferiority complex in the child and many other complications. He will then begin to stammer more.

- **Support from other children**

Support from other children and co-students increases the self-confidence in the child who stammers. Teachers can prompt and motivate the child to read aloud in class. Other students too should not imitate or ridicule this child for his stammer. If the child stammers or stutters, the teacher can ask the child to read the lesson/page at home and repeat it in the class the next day again.

- **Impartial behaviour**

The teachers should be impartial in their behaviour. If the child who stammers has a behavioural problem, then the teacher should try to help him. The teacher too likes parents can build self-confidence in the child so that the child can speak out his problem or complaint in front of the teacher.

As a conclusion it can be said that the child having a

stammering problem should be treated like normal children both at home and school. The child should not get a feeling that people are sympathetic towards him or acting out of pity because this can have an adverse impact on him.

Parents should try to take initiative to rectify the problem as soon as it comes to their notice. It is fairly easy to treat this problem in a child of 8-9 years, whereas it may consume a lot of time if the child is over 15 years of age. The child himself can get over this problem with his firm determination.

It is mandatory to consult a speech therapist if the problem has turned grave.

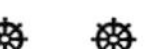

16

UNWILLINGNESS TO GO TO SCHOOL

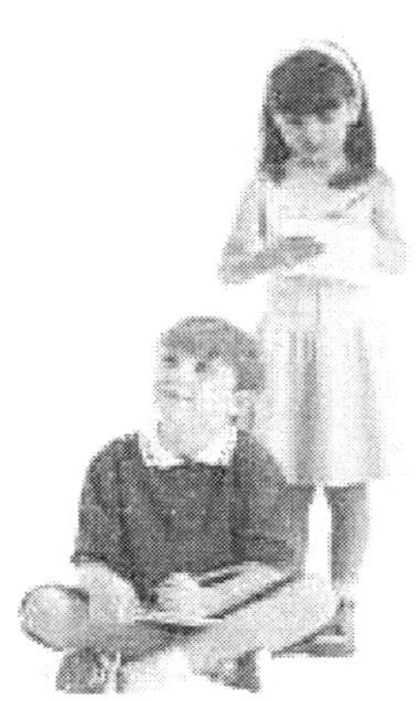

By the time the child reaches the age of 3-4 years parents are haunted by the thought of sending their young ones to a good school. This situation is a very traumatic one for both the children and the parents. Initially the parents get the child into a nearby neighbourhood playschool to familiarise him with the relatively new school going routine. Thereafter the parents start looking for a bigger, better school for the child. Some children adjust to the new system quite happily and willingly. New schoolbag, attractive water bottles and tiffin box add to their happiness. Such children befriend other children quickly. Most children move into the process naturally. However, some children start hesitating to go to the school as soon as the fancy for the new things begins to wear off. They start crying and throwing a fit at the time of school in such a way that the entire school going exercise appears to be a punishment.

There are some children who begin crying from day one. It is normal and quite natural for young children to cry while going to school initially. They are going to enter an unfamiliar environment from a cocoon of love and security. They settle down gradually with passage of time.

If a child aged 4-5 years or above cries or hesitates to go to school or if a child who has been going to school quite normally for years suddenly starts showing an unwillingness towards going to school, then it is worthwhile to investigate the reasons behind this. There can be many reasons behind the unwillingness to go to school. Parents should try to talk to the child about why he doesn't wish to go to school, instead of forcibly sending them to school day after day despite his total unwillingness. If the child is between 12-15 years of age (of either sex) and hesitates in going to schools, and still you are continuing to send him to school, without finding the cause of his hesitation can sometimes lead to grave consequences like, the child leaving home altogether or even committing suicide.

Most parents either scold or beat the child in order to send him to school forcibly. This way the child will go to school out of the fear of his parents despite not wishing to go school out of the fear of his parents despite not wishing to go and his problems and inhibitions keep troubling him, as he is unable to discuss them with his parents. His dilemma brings about abnormal changes in his behaviour and he starts losing his self-confidence.

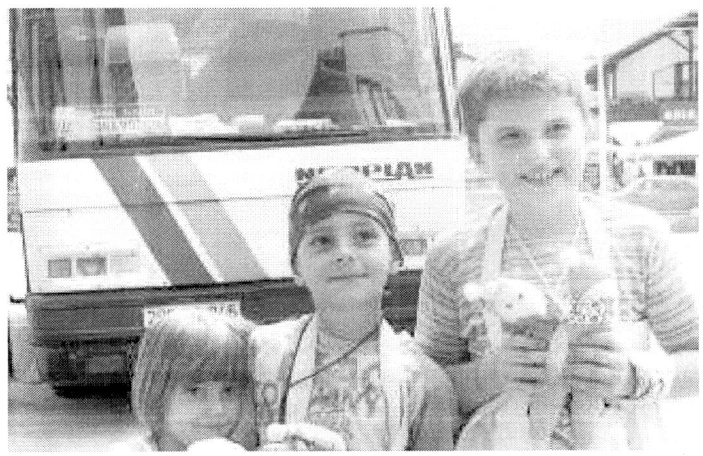

CAUSES AND SOLUTIONS

If the child expresses his unwillingness to go to school on an everyday basis, try to make him open up about the issue rather than sending him to school forcibly or by promising rewards etc. The child may be hesitating from going to school because of the following reasons:

- **Inability to fulfil the expectations of the parents**

It is the desire of every parent to see their child coming first or securing higher grades in school. However, some children are unable to fare well in studies and are scared to show their marks to their parents. They feel if they can avoid going to school altogether, they can escape this entire quagmire of studies and marks. These thoughts motivate children to start avoiding going to school.

Solutions

If the child is avoiding school because he is unable to come first in his class, then parents should first understand themselves and also explain to the child that not every child can come first in his class. Parents should encourage their child to work hard and perform to the best of his ability. Parents should feel satisfied if the child is doing his best even if he is not getting highest marks.

- **Tension and unpleasantness between parents**

If there is tension and differences of opinion between the parents in the family, the child starts to feel insecure. He fears that he might spell out the problems at home unconsciously to his classmates or teachers at school and might become a laughing stock before everyone.

Solutions

The parents have to ensure that no situation of arguments or tension arises in front of the child. In case the child is aware of the situation at home, parents should work towards developing his self confidence so that he is able to counter all pleasant and unpleasant situations boldly.

- **The teacher's incorrect teaching method**

Some teachers teach in a manner that all students are not able to understand the lesson. Intelligent students understand the chapter with their own efforts, whereas those who have an average I.Q. are unable to understand the same. When these students approach the teacher to solve their problems, the teacher too is unable to satisfy their query of the child and often scolds the child for being inattentive etc. Thus such students hesitate from going to the school for fear of punishment, scolding etc.

Solutions

Parents should first enquire about the reasons for hesitation from the child and then go and meet the concerned teacher or the headmistress. In addition to this, they should take interest in the child's studies and also motivate him to self-study.

- **Discriminatory and rude behaviour of the teacher**

Some teachers prefer smart and intelligent students over other students and pay more attention towards them. Sometimes they become prejudiced against a particular child and punish or scold the child for small mistakes also. The child dreads the idea of going to school out of fear of the teacher. Sometimes such teachers corner the child with difficult questions so that they can punish "the particular child" if he fails to give an answer. These teachers also give corporal punishments to the children which scare away the children from the idea of school altogether.

Solutions

First and foremost try to find out the cause of the problems that is, what actions or mistakes of the child irritates or angers the teacher and ask the child to avoid repeating the same in the future.

Parents should also approach the teacher concerned and try to solve the problems of the child by amicable discussions. If many children in the class are facing a similar problem, then it is best to meet the principal of the school for the problem.

Teachers too, should adopt an impartial behaviour towards all students and should keep away from giving very strict and corporal punishments to the children. Corporal punishments never have any positive effect on the academic performance of the child.

Teachers should have a balanced and sympathetic behaviour towards all students. They should try to first try to find out the reason why the child has done his mistake or is inattentive in class before taking recourse to punishments. Unnecessary punishments and scolding should be avoided.

- **Physical handicap (disability) or low mental I.Q. of the child**

Physical handicap in a child of any form creates a low self-esteem or self-confidence in the child. In such a situation if he is ridiculed at school and the teacher doesn't adopt a sympathetic behaviour towards the child, he doesn't want to go to school.

Solutions

Parents should inculcate loads self-confidence in their child and develop courage to face and counter his disability.

If the child complains that the other students are making fun of him at school, then the parents should meet the teacher concerned immediately. In any case parents should brief the teacher concerned about the problem of the child so that she/he can be empathetic towards the child.

The teachers too should adopt a sympathetic and understanding behaviour towards children with disabilities and those with a low I.Q. They should try to make other children too adapt to these children and keep all the children as a group.

- **If the child has more inclinations towards games than studies**

Some children are naturally more inclined towards sports than studies and do not show much interest in studies. Consequently they find the idea of going to school unacceptable and unpalatable.

Solutions

Such children pose to be a great problem for the parents as teachers constantly keep complaining about these children. Parents should explain the importance of studies to the children. If the child wishes to adopt sports as a career, then parents should be supportive of that, but also motivate him to pursue studies side by side.

- **Not able to get along with other children or bullying by other children**

If the child is more than 12 years of age and is unwilling or hesitant to go to school, then parents should take the matter seriously and try to find out the reasons behind it. It is quite possible that the child has picked up a quarrel with other students or is a victim of bullying by senior students etc.

There can also be interpersonal problems between boys and girls in co-educational schools, which can be a deterrent in going to school.

Solutions

Parents have to find out the problem and a solution too at their end only. Sending the child forcibly can complicate matters and can make the child be averse towards studies as well.

There can be many such reasons for the child showing disinterest in going to school. Some of these can be like this: other children forcibly snatching the child's tiffin, other children sitting on his seat, bullying by other children etc. Parents should handle the problem according to the gravity of the problem. Do not force the child to succumb to your order and forcibly send him to school. Try to find a solution to his problem first.

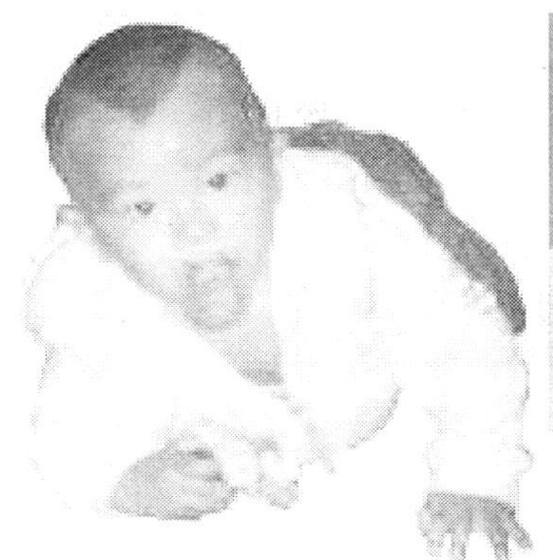

17 SHORT-TEMPEREDNESS

Many children start exhibiting their anger overtly by either shouting or by throwing things here and there when they want elders to succumb to their wishes or when they want to pull attention towards them. Some children on the other hand, express their anger when they find themselves lonely or when they are suffering from an inferiority complex.

Let us see Rahul"s example. Whenever guests come over to pay them a visit, six year old Rahul starts throwing things all over the place in anger because as his mother starts attending to the guests and many times doesn't listen to him. Rahul feels neglected and lonely. On the other hand Saurabh starts crying aloud whenever he feels angry about something.

Whatever the reason, if your child is prone to be short tempered, then it is in his interest to teach him to control his temper or else he will end up being extremely obstinate and undisciplined as he grows up. Also he will never be able to cultivate normal relationships with others as he grows older. It is possible that he is not able to carry good relationship with his spouse after marriage only because of his short temperedness.

Generally speaking, anger is a fairly normal and natural emotion, which is experienced by both adults and children, though in varying degrees. But if children are not taught to control their anger from the correct age, then one can face harsh consequences for the same as they grow.

As parents it is but natural for you to be tolerant towards your child's anger, but that doesn't mean that he/she will be equally tolerated by others as well for behaviour such as shrieking, breaking objects etc. in a fit of anger. If the child forms a habit out of expressing his anger in a destructive way, he will behave in a similar manner before others as well. If the child is allowed to behave in this way, he will start moving in the direction of violence and if parents are unable to curtail their child in this regard, then they can be rest assured about leading the child towards a dark future.

It is not necessary that children acquire a temper at the age of 5-7 years. Sometimes it so happens that normal and soft-natured children too begin to get short tempered as they start moving towards adolescence. They vent out their anger at their parents or whoever is vulnerable to them and then start using them to accept all their wishes and demands. Normally children become short-tempered at the toddler stage or after they enter their teenage. The age between the above two ages, i.e. from 7-8 years is the time when their temperaments are more or less child like. However, parents should exercise control over the child whenever he loses temper.

Ill-Effects of Anger

Anger is no doubt a very negative emotion and it has negative effects on everyone. According to psychologists, anger affects both the body and the mind of an individual. Anger can result in the following negative consequences as far as child is concerned:

- A short tempered child tends to be naughty and obstinate.
- If parents continue to put up with this temperament of the child, he begins to move further in the direction of violence.
- If this feeling of anger is allowed to dwell in child in his childhood stage, then anger becomes a part and parcel of his personality (his habits and behaviour), which eventually has an effect on the social life of the child after he grows up.
- The ill effects of anger become evident in his physical and mental self as he grows up.
- Short-tempered children are unable to form a relationship after they grow up and they are also not able to enjoy a peaceful and normal family life.
- If this negative emotion is not controlled at the right time it hampers the career of the child as well when he grows up. He is unable to keep normal relations with anyone in the office e.g. his boss or colleagues.
- Extremely short-tempered children often throw things here and there in anger. Such an action results in unnecessary damage of household items (and therefore financial loses) and can cause an injury to others as well.
- Short-tempered children also tend to use foul and unparliamentary language as they grow a little older and earn the tag of "indecent and undisciplined child" subsequently.

MEASURES TO CONTROL THE CHILD'S TEMPER

First and foremost parents should understand and accept anger as a natural process. In today's times when tension and stress cause anger in adults, children too can become a victim of the same. However, extreme short temper can prove to be harmful for the child. This is when they need to be counseled and guided in the proper direction so that they can control the temper.

- If the child is expressing his anger in a destructive way, then he should be slowly told the difference between violent anger and normal emotion of anger.
- Parents should not give in to all the demands of the child if he is being extremely short tempered or obstinate over a demand. The child should be made to understand the difference between right and wrong from the beginning itself.
- Parents should never vent out their personal anger on their kids. Children suppress this anger within them and express it at some point later.
- One should control one's temper first. Do not use foul words, violence, insult etc. for in front of your children as these things will find their way into the child's conscience as well.
- In anger never behave in a way that will make you repent or regret. Try to express your anger in a decent way.
- If you see that your child is angry, give him an opportunity to speak out the cause and try to understand his behaviour. Do not start beating him or punishing in any other way then you see him in anger before listening to him.
- Explain the difference between good and bad behaviour at leisure time. Guide and direct him to take right decisions at the right time.
- Do not scold or ridicule the child in front of his friends as this makes him feel insulted which he will express later in the form of anger.

- Do not order the child at all times. Be a friend to him too. Play with him, talk to him whenever you get an opportunity so that the child too can relieve his tensions with you.
- Be strict with the child if he expresses his anger in a wrong way. Leniency in the initial stages can reinforce this into a bad habit and make him short-tempered.
- If you keep fulfilling all the demands of the child, whether right or wrong, he becomes used to it. At a later stage if you want to put your foot down to any of his demands, he is unable to digest it and starts resorting to throwing / breaking things etc; to know his displeasure and anger. Therefore always follow a right and balanced approach.
- If you have hit the child for any reason, then as soon as the phase subsides, express your love to the child. This will make the child feel loved and protected and he will understand that it was his mistake that prompted you to act in a strict manner with him. He will know that your anger too was momentary and you love him very much otherwise.
- Be patient and calm even when the child does something wrong. This will teach him to control his anger as well. Scold him lightly or make him understand his mistake in a calm tone. Remember, you are his role model.
- Love your child unconditionally and tell him about the negative consequences of anger so that child moves in the right direction in life and becomes an ideal citizen when he grows up.

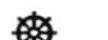

18

THE HABIT OF LYING

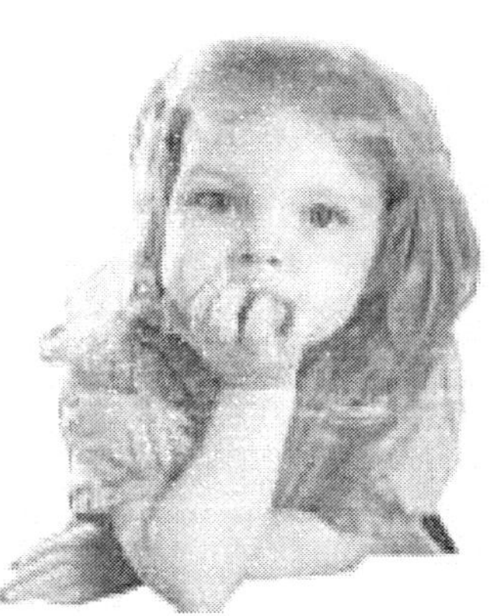

Mihir was the darling of his family. But he had one bad habit – the habit of lying. One day, Mihir happened to break a flower-vase. He went inside his room and set down to study as if nothing was happened. After a while his mother came home and was horrified and angry on seeing the expensive flower-vase broken. When she asked Mihir about it, he feigned innocence about the vase and said he had been in his room studying for a long time. Mihir's mother started to reprimand the maid-servant without hearing her out. Mihir of course was very very happy and relieved that he had escaped from the act because of his lie. Slowly and gradually Mihir started becoming a compulsive liar.

Many children lie for each and everything. They have a ready excuse for not completing their homework; they lie to their parents also for the same. They keep looking for and invent lies for everything. This habit of lying becomes so bad that people start disbelieving them even if they say the truth. At times they are punished or scolded even when they speak the truth. The consequences of this habit of lying have to be borne by them.

Children who lie too much eventually turn out to be crooks

or cheats. They try to prove themselves to be smart and intelligent, but eventually the truth comes out one day or the other.

WHY DOES A CHILD LIE?

Initially the child lies just for fun – hiding a small thing like a pencil or a handkerchief and saying that a crow has taken it – everybody laughs at these incidents. But over the years, unable to differentiate between right and wrong, the child starts lying even for small things.

The child starts picking up the habit of lying from his home – from his parents, grandparents, uncle, aunt, maid, servant or any other member of his family. For e.g.: when the children is taken to a doctor for an injection, he is told that it will not be painful – but it actually is – and he realises that his parents had lied to him when they brought him to the doctor. Lying to him had made their task easier. Thus, with this small lie starts the child's inclination towards lie and also his mistrust you.

Many small (and seemingly insignificant) lies that parents resort to in front of the child – evoke a deep sense of distrust in the child's mind. Harmless lies – which are always taken for granted, too have their impact on the child. Sometimes the child is promised a reward – if he gets good marks – which is never fulfilled even after the success or the mother promising the child to be back in an hour but comes after 5-6 hours. All these small things create sense mistrust in the child's mind about his parents and he too resorts to lying. Another example is if the father wishes to avoid a certain phone call and asks the child to lie that he (father) is not at home. These affect the child deeply and he also takes recourse to lying. Some children learn it from their servants inadvertently or even from their friends. What starts playfully, initially – gradually becomes a compulsive habit – the habit of lying.

Lying is a bad habit. The child loses his credibility Because of this habit. He is able to hide all his other bad habits in the garb of his lies. Sometimes it is to late when everything comes out in the open. Because of this habit of lying – the child learns to steal, lags behind in his studies and gets caught in many other related problems.

Children can learn to lie in any age – whether he is five or fifteen. Grown up children lie to their parents about smoking or drinking habits or even driving a two-wheeler or cars. Adolescent children generally pick up this habit of lying from their friends. Their friends instigate them to lie for many things.

HOW TO RECTIFY THE HABIT OF LYING

1. First and foremost children should be inspired to speak only the truth. The habit of lying in a child should not be taken lightly. He should be taught the negative consequences of lies and the importance of truth.
2. If the child fears punishments – scolding or beating on speaking the truth, then he resorts to telling lies. Try to elicit the truth from the child tactfully and lovingly – don't start beating him immediately when he does something wrong, otherwise he will always tell lies to avoid punishment.
3. Try to listen to the child's view point when he goes wring so that he doesn't resort to telling lies.
4. Repeatedly make the child realise about the difference between truth and lie. Make him understand how harmful

it is to resort to lying in order to escape from beating or scolding.

5. Try to be truthful to the child. Tell the child that it is necessary to have an injection to his ailment and it will be a little painful – but it is for his own good.

6. If the child demands an expensive item which you cannot afford – tell him the truth it is too costly for you to afford it. Instead of criticising the item, try to convince the child and satisfy him.

7. Don't lie in front of the child time and again. Lies told at home on a daily basis which seem fairly harmless can leave a deep impact on the child's mind. If the mother lies to the father or vice versa, this encourages the child too to tell lies. If the mother wants to hide something and tells the child also not to speak up in front of the father, then next time the child will lie to his mother when he does something wrong. There should be transparency in the behaviour of the father and mother.

8. If the child starts lying too much then strict measures can be adopted to correct him.

9. Don't side with the child when he lies in front of his teacher or any other member of the family. To safeguard him don't defend the child by lying when he lies. This will encourage him to lie and also force you lie.

Right from his initial stage, make the child realise the ill effects of lying and importance of truth, to save him from becoming a liar. Also, prepare him to face the situations – good or bad in his life with equal courage and confidence.

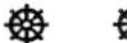

19

HYPERACTIVITY IN CHILDREN

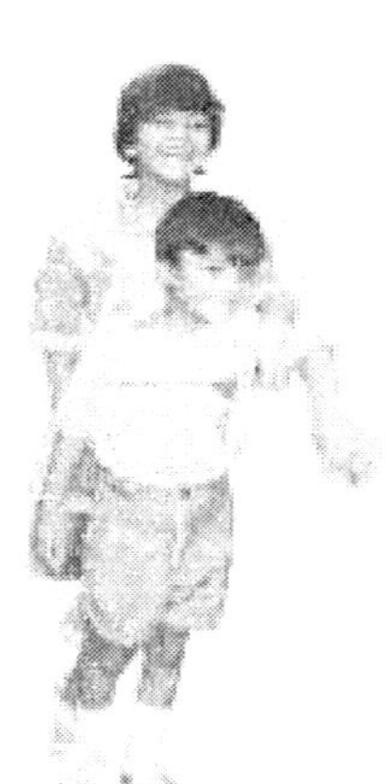

Now-a-days generally children are quite smart and extremely active. These are the children, of today's modern – fast moving world, intelligent and smart from the time they come into this world, quite capable of understanding everything in no time. These are not our times anymore.

But some of these children are over-active. They can never sit at one place; they keep running here and there and are unable to concentrate on one single task. If a task is given to them, which is of there liking, they finish it in minutes, which would have otherwise taken hours. Such children can neither sit in peace themselves nor do they allow their parents to be in peace. Such children are known as hyperactive children.

Hyperactive children never like to do things for which they will have to sit in one place. Even if such a task is given to them they try to do finish it as fast as possible. They don't even bother to see if it has been done properly, they merely want to finish it. People who are observing them feel as if they are in an urgency to go out somewhere that is why they are finishing their work in a hurry.

In today's world hyperactive children can be found in every

second or third household. When the child is around 3-4 years old and at home one can enjoy his hyper activeness. But once he starts growing and is unable to concentrate on anything whether it is his studies, sports or any other work involving responsibility, then he starts becoming a troublesome to the parents.

Generally parents think that the child is extremely mischievous and he therefore is unable to concentrate on his studies. When he sit down to study, he keeps finding excuses to get up like to have a glass of water, to get a pen or pencil from the next room etc. According to child specialist Dr. S. Sethi, in scientific terminology this situation is called, "Hyperactive Disorder". Somewhat similar to this is another problem which is known as, "Attention Deficient Disorder".

Kabir's teacher used to said repeated complaints to his parents to come and meet her. Every time they meet the teacher, they were told - Kabir doesn't sit at one place, doesn't listen to instructions and is very mischievous. If he is scolded, he sits for two minutes and then starts his activities all over again, would want to visit the toilet, what is his problem?"

Kabir frequently used to get negative marking; sometimes his note-books carried warning remarks also. But he never changed and remained the same restless boy. When his parents took him to a child psychologist they were told by him that Kabir suffered from scientific problem which is known as "Attention Deficient Hyper Active Disorder." Such children possess more energy level as compared to normal children, so they spend their extra energy in running around.

Symptoms

- Hyperactive children are extremely restless. They cannot

sit quietly in one place. They hate doing any type of work sitting at one place. They like to run here and there and do their work. Such children never sit peacefully.

- They want to try any new thing given to them on their own with their own hands. They first open and scrutinise a new toy or any other new thing that is given to them instead of playing with it. This way their toys (particularly the ones that are operated by keys) become useless very soon.
- Such children are highly energetic if any relative or any acquaintance wants to talk to them, instead of standing still a few minutes and talking with them, they are always on the move when they are talking. Their energy level is so high that if they are assigned any task involving going up and down or running around, the task is finished in no time by them.
- Hyperactive children are generally very talkative. Therefore, they invent a long story to say one simple thing. If they want to say something that happened at the school, a matter of one minute will take 5-10 minutes, even if they have to add things on their own.
- Hyperactive children are generally very inquisitive and therefore ask lots of questions – like why it happens, how it happens, etc. often they spend their entire energy in asking meaningless questions.
- Hyperactive children feel less hungry or it may be said that because of their restlessness they find it difficult to sit at one place and finish their food. It may also be possible that some hyperactive children feel hungrier than others. Their extra energy is wasted in mischief, running around etc. so they feel more hungry. Nevertheless, whether they

feel less hungry or more hungry, they cannot sit peacefully at one place and eat their food. They eat a little while they are playing or running here and there, then when the mother beckons them to have food, they eat some more. This is how they eat their food.

- Hyperactive children feel happier in disrupting a game rather than playing it. They are always in a hurry to be on the forefront. They cannot let others play peacefully. They play on their own terms – if they are made the captain and everybody listens to them, then the game goes on peacefully. Otherwise they have no patience to wait for their turn and soon disturb/destroy the whole game.
- It is generally seen that such children lack patience. If you assign them any work, without waiting to listen to the whole thing – they run off or else they say – 'tell me fast' – I have to do this work or my friend is waiting for me or I am going to miss my TV programme etc. Due to lack of patience, they are in a hurry to tell what they want to say and also want other to be fast when they talk, even though they have an urge to exaggerate their story to make it longer. Due to this lack of patience only, they try to reply in the least possible words, if any relative or acquaintance tries to talk to them. Else, they escape from that place saying that he/she will be back soon.
- Hyperactive children generally sleep less. After coming back from school, instead of resting or relaxing, they indulge in mischief. Many a times, it so happens that in an effort to put the child to sleep, the mother dozes off while the child silently slips from the bed and busies himself in playing.

REASONS AND DIFFICULTIES

According to Dr. S. Sethi there are two main reasons for hyperactivity in children. First is hereditary and second is by birth and bodily chemical changes. These chemical charges are known as Dopaoni chemicals. Because of this chemical only, the child's mind is not stable and he keeps doing mischief. On the first sight there appear to be no obvious problems due to the child being hyperactive.

But due to their extreme restlessness as they are unable to concentrate on their studies so they don't do well. Such as child is so mischievous that sometimes he creates difficulties not only for others but ends up hurting himself also at times.

Nevertheless, hyperactive children are quite intelligent, though because of their impatience they don't listen to others and like to have to their own way. Many a times, they make up tall tales to short work.

If, they get negative remarks from the school due to their mischievous nature, then inferiority complex starts developing in these children. If a proper solution is not found to this problem of hyperactive children, then there is a possibility that they start losing their self-confidence.

Such children get scolded both by parents and their teachers. They fail to understand their mistakes and develop a rebellious attitude. They think that if they do something wrong then they get so much scolding and beating but if some other child does this nobody says anything. The fact is that other children show this type of behaviour only very rarely.

As these children don't eat properly and adequately, they are not healthy and strong and tend to be very thin physically. The parents of course want them to be healthy but they remain very thin.

These children try to escape from their studies as they are more involved in doing mischief and idle talks. Because of their unstable mind, sometimes they are unable to take right decisions, as well.

SOLUTIONS

An active and a naughty kid is liked by all but only upto a limit. For this parents can certain seek medical help, now-a days and also get counselling done from child psychologists.

Child guidance centres /clinics in cities give proper guidance to parents on how to improve these children tactfully, in an appropriate manner.

In the counselling sessions, apart from the parents, children are also given training on how to control themselves in different situations. In order to improve the behaviour of hyperactive children, the cooperation of the school and teacher is must.

Medical science tries to treat such children with the help of different drugs. Sleep inducing tablets (sedatives) are prescribed to make them sleep well, which gives them less time to indulge in mischief. But generally parents are not very keen to use medicines, which slow down the child. They believe that these medicines may prove harmful to the children in the longer run.

SUGGESTIONS ON BEHAVIOUR

Certain behavioural suggestions can be brought into use for hyperactive children.

- Because of their enormous energy level, the extra energy can be put to some constructive use. Keeping in mind the taste or talent of the child he can be motivated to make artistic things. If the child is interested in sports, he can be given formal training in any game of his choice.

- The child's confidence and patience level improves if he is entrusted with some responsibility, e.g. he can assigned the responsibility of looking after his younger sister or brother, dusting or clearing his table or keeping his bed clean.
- If the child doesn't eat well – instead of giving him something every now and then it would be better if he is fed when he is very hungry so that he eats a full hearty meal. Don't try to tempt the child in between with chocolates or other tit-bits. Eating snacks in between meals suppresses his hunger and makes the child eat very less food.
- If the child asks intelligent questions, don't be afraid to give him the right answer and increase his knowledge. Thus in his class also he will be known as an intelligent child.
- If he is over-talkative try to make him understand the uselessness of such talk. With time, he will learn to talk sensibly.
- Try to build up his patience and confidence. He may also be advised to put up good behaviour while playing with other children.

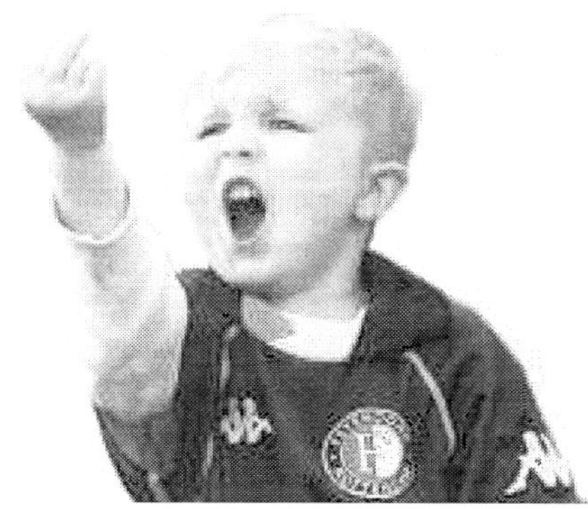

20

IRRITABILITY

In this time and age of tension and pressure, irritability, jealousy and competitive feelings are increasing in our society, so they are found in the children as well. The problems of irritability can be found in a child of any age – from an infant to an adolescent.

Let us primarily understand the concept of irritability first. 'Irritability" is a situation when a child or a teenager gets miffed unnecessarily and without any important reason. In the process he harms himself in his bed temper at times and at other times he vents out his anger on his parents or other family members. An infant cries time and again out of his irritability. If a 6-7 months old infant cries persistently, it is often said that the child is perhaps irritable (probably because he is teething or may be he has any problem somewhere.)

Along with the child himself, his parents too suffer similarly the consequences of untimely anger and irritability. The child's constant irritability begins to affect his academic performance as well and he starts lagging behind in his class. Tension and pressures of different kinds aggravate the feeling of irritability in the child.

Ruchi called her nine-year old daughter Sunaina, "Darling, will you come here for a minute?" Sunaina resorted back, "I am coming ma, why you don't wait?" and went to her mother seething with anger. This often happens.

CAUSES

Upbringing of the child is a very important factor behind any negative behaviour of a child. Apart from upbringing, there are other important causes as well. The following causes can attribute to irritability:

- **Repeated nagging**

Raima's mother had a habit of nagging Raima at each and every instance. Raima too never retaliated and did everything according to her mother till she was about 7-8 years old. But as she began to grow older, she began to get irritated at her mother's constant nagging and interference. If she was watching T.V., her mother would want her to sit down to study. When she would start making notes, her mother would ask her to concentrate on learning as well and not just go on scribbling. In this manner Raima's mother commented on each and every action of hers. Gradually Raima turned into an irritable child because of her mother's nagging attitude. Thus constant interference and nagging can turn a normal child into an obstinate or irritable child.

These days, children engage a lot in telephonic conversations for long hours. On being enquired and advised about the same by the parents, children often turn irritable and lose their temper as well at small instances.

- **Extreme academic pressure**

When the child is under a lot of pressure for his studies, especially when the examination are fast approaching and the child has not completed his preparation, he is likely to get irritable. This situation is more pronounced with class 10th or 12th students, when they have a burden of their parents expectations along with their own apprehension and pressure. Unable to cope with pressure from all sides, they end up getting extremely irritable.

- **Repeated comparison**

If a child is constantly compared with his classmates or other children, he begins to feel angry and the same finds an expression in his irritability. Some children find some comparisons irksome and emphasise that they are completely different from the other child and do not like to be compared. When exams results were declared Sudhanshu's father called him and said, "Sudhanshu, why have you scored such low marks this time? Why don't you learn something from your brother Priyanshu? See how well he's done." This comparison turned Sudhanshu green with jealousy and in a fit of anger as he began sharpening his pencil with a knife; he cut his finger as well. In this situation even though the father was very much right in what he said, he could have well avoided the comparison, which had a totally undesired effect on the child. Children begin to feel insulted at being compared with a sibling or friends time and again and display irritability when the action is repeated.

- **Incomplete / inadequate sleep**

Child of any age is bound to get irritable if he does not take adequate quantity of sleep. 5 year old Kritika cried everyday when she was woken up to go to school. Her mother could never understand that lack of sleep was making her behave in this manner. She thought Kritika was doing all this to avoid school.

- **Contradictory behaviour**

If a child is reprimanded for an action one day and praised for the same on another day, he is unable to take a decision about right and wrong. On being scolded unreasonably at different occasions, he becomes irritable. Whenever Abhay used to show his test notebook to his mother, she used to brush it off and asked how much Abhay's classmate Anshu had scored in the test. Abhay said. "Mamma, Anshu always cheats in all the tests. He has scored better than me." His father who was listening to this conversation interrupted, "Good marks are all that matters, the means are immaterial."

In the next test, Abhay too attempted to cheat and was caught red-handed by the teacher. When his parents were informed about the same, Abhay was taken to ask severely. His father scolded him and said. "Why did you cheat? Get whatever marks you can at your own merit." Abhay didn't know to react.

Similarly at many occasions when there are fights at school and parents learn about it, sometimes they ask the child not to fight back, while at other times they themselves ask the child not to be timid and hit the other child in his defence.

These types of contradictory orders confuse the child and make him irritable too.

- **Over imposition on the child**

Everyday child wants to prove himself on the basis of his capability. However if the parents keep imposing their views on the child and want him to act according to their directions always and do not appreciate the child's individual effort, he is bound to get irritable.

SOLUTIONS

Children need to be given proper guidance from parents, guardians and teachers so that irritability can be kept at bay. Also parents should have complete understanding and harmony so that they do not give contradictory instructions to the child, which will impart an ideal personality to the child. One of the parents should always know and support the same cause, whatever the other has instructed. There should contradiction between parents' statements.

Paying attention to the following things can help to prevent irritability in the child.

- Do not pressurise the child to study more than he can.
- If he feels tensed or stressed because of his studies, talk to him and try to ease his stress. Make the child take small breaks in between studies to break the monotony and relieve stress as well.
- Prepare a TV and study schedule for the child so that he doesn't have to be reminded to study (which can be irritating for him) time and again.
- Do not impose your thoughts on your child every time. Cultivate the habit of responsible decision making in him.
- If parents spend 'quality time" with the child, i.e. they talk to the child and play or engage in other meaningful activities, it can develop a greater understanding between the two and the child is less likely to be irritable.
- Know your child's desires and interests. Guide him to pursue studies and games accordingly.
- Develop a feeling in the child that the child is extremely important to you and matters the most. Whenever he appears stressed or tensed, discuss the situation on a 'one

to one basis" with him and then try to help him get out of it.

- Never compare a child with his friends or siblings. Every child is unique in his own way. Some children excel in games and some in creative pursuits.
- Make the child aware of the difference between the right and the wrong. But avoid imposing your ideology on him.
- Let the child be himself. Do not force him to imitate or try to be someone else.
- Do not give a free hand to the child in everything. It is right to impose restrictions on the child in some matters.
- Make a definite time table for the child for sleeping and waking up from the very beginning so that he gets used to the same. Incomplete sleep leaves the child irritable.
- Do not keep nagging the child for each and everything. He should be scolded and questioned only if he commits a mistake.
- Respect the child's opinion while discussing different options for a gift to be purchased for any child. Do not ignore his suggestion first because he is a kid. Listen to it carefully and accept it if it suits the occasion. This boosts the child's self-confidence.

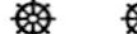

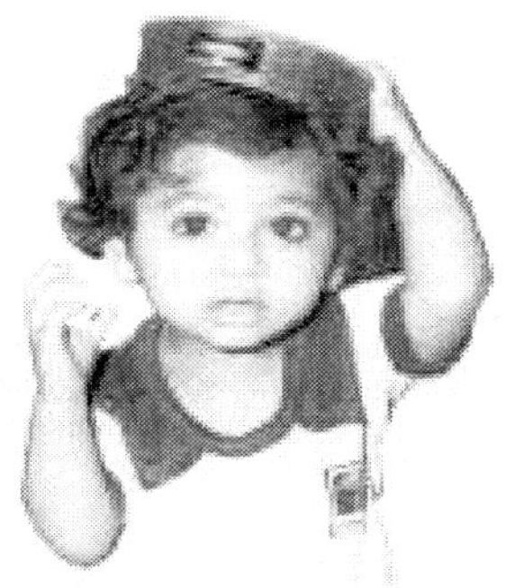

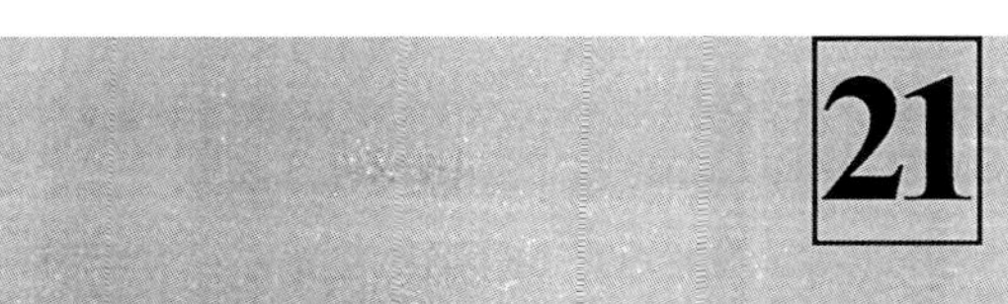

21 SLEEPLESSNESS (INSOMNIA)

Many parents keep complaining about the inadequate or improper sleep of their children. Some children do not sleep peacefully the whole night because of which they appear to be tired and drained out the next day.

According to child psychologist Dr. Hardip, "Lack of sleep affects the growth process in a child. Adequate sleep is a must for sound health." He has advised the following sleep schedule for children according to their age:

AGE		EXPECTED SLEEP TIME
3 Months - 1 Year	:-	14-15 hours
1 Year - 3 Years	:-	12-14 hours
3 Year - 6 Years	:-	11-12 hours
6 Year - 12 Years	:-	10-11 hours
12 year - 18 Years	:-	8½-9½ hours
Average individuals	:-	8 hours

Doctors are of the belief that children who do not get adequate sleep during the day do not have a sound memory as compared to those who sleep adequately. Such children also succumb to common ailments like cough, cold and other communicable diseases very soon. Sleeplessness (insomnia) reduces a person's ability to acquire/assimilate information and working capacity.

For children of all ages adequate sleep is as important as proper diet. Complete sleep plays a vital role in keeping the child active and mentally healthy. In the morning the child gets up fresh. A child with good sleep habits results in giving the child a proper focus and gives a good memory power to him. Dr. Hardip believes that "a child's physical ability and the ability to focus remains very good if he gets good sleep during the nights."

Consequent Problems

If the child doesn't get his complete sleep or is a victim of insomnia, the following problems can crop up as well:

- If a child has not been getting complete sleep, he tends to become irritable.
- Incomplete sleep makes the child feel tired and exhausted and affects his day-to-day activities.
- Incomplete sleep drains the child of his energy and enthusiasm because of which he is unable to show an interest towards games and other such activities.
- If the child has not slept properly the previous night, he tends to doze off during class hours.
- Adequate sleep makes the child irritable towards going to school the next day.
- The child becomes more susceptible towards cold, fever and other communicable diseases.
- The child tends to oversleep into the day to compensate

for his incomplete sleep, which makes him lose out on other activities of the day.

- The child can suffer from headaches.
- Eyes appear tired and heavy on account of inadequate sleep.
- If a person is a victim of insomnia from his childhood, his under-eye becomes swollen, dark and heavy. His eyesight can also be adversely affected and he may be forced to wear spectacles.
- The child is unable to concentrate on one thing because of incomplete sleep. He feels extremely tired and sick.

CAUSES FOR INADEQUATE SLEEP

• Improper sleep routine

If the child does not go to sleep at fixed time and keeps chatting with his family members or watches TV late into the night, he is unable to get his share of sleep, which subsequently leads to many other problems as well.

• Sleeping during the day for long hours

Montu's mother put him to sleep as soon as he came back from school and finished his lunch. He slept for 3-4 hours at a stretch (sometimes till 7-8 P.M.) as his mother did not like to wake him up. The result was that he didn't sleep till 12 o' clock in the night because of his sleep during the day and troubled his parents as well. Again he could not get his complete sleep as he had slept late.

Once or twice his mother saw Montu watching an adult's movie at about 1 or 2 A.M. when his mother questioned him about it, he said simply that he was not feeling sleepy and when he switched on T.V., only this movie was coming in the T.V.

Therefore, sleeping more during the daytime can result in negative consequences.

- **Father coming late from work**

Businessmen or people working in multinational companies have long working hours and often return home very late. As the child goes off to school early morning and is unable to meet the father, as the father gets up late, the mother keeps the child awake late in the night so that he can meet his father at night. The result is that child is not able to take adequate sleep.

- **Tensed atmosphere at home**

If unpleasantness and quarrels are rampant in the house atmosphere, the child's psyche gets adversely affected by the same and he often gets up in the middle of the night scared. He is unable to sleep peacefully if this happens on regular basis.

- **No sleep during the daytime**

If the child engages in games or homework etc. after coming back from school and doesn't sleep at all in the day and the mother doesn't motivate the child to sleep early in the night too, then his sleep remains incomplete. If the child doesn't sleep during the day, then he must be put to sleep by 7-8 in the night.

- **Studying late night**

If the child is studying in middle or secondary classes (class VI onwards) and studies late night, he is unable to complete his sleep. In such a situation he falls asleep in the class.

TIPS FOR SOUND SLEEP

- Make a sleep schedule for the child. Even if the elders in the family have a habit of sleeping late, make sure that the child sleeps early at an appropriate time. Let him have his dinner at the right time. Then at the prescribed time dim his room lights and put him to sleep.

- Do not allow the child to watch T.V. at night.
- Allot time for the child for his specific tasks during the day. Learn the art of 'Time Management' so that child can study, play and sleep in the right quantity.
- If the child sleeps at the right time everyday and wishes to stay awake for one day in a week to spend more time and enjoy with his family, he can be allowed to do so.
- Keep the child engaged in various activities throughout the day so that he consumes his energy and feels tired and sleeps soundly at night. If all he does throughout the day sit in front of the T.V. or computer, then he may not be able to get sound sleep.
- Make the child sleep for 1-2 hours after he comes back from school so that he wakes up refreshed.
- If the child insists to sleep more during the day, persuade him gently to get up and engage him in the activities he likes.
- If the child doesn't sleep at all during the day, make sure that sleeps at 7-8 P.M. at night.
- It would be ideal to cultivate "Early to bed early to rise" habit in the child so that he sleeps and gets up on time. This is key to perfect health.
- Keeps the child away from stress and tension so that he sleeps in a relaxed manner.
- Do not pressurize the child to study. If the child keeps studying late into the night is under great pressure, he is unable to sleep properly.

- If the child listens to a lullaby, bedtime story or soothing music for sometime before sleeping, he is likely to sleep more soundly.
- Have a soothing night bulb in the child's room so that the child doesn't wake up scared and is able to complete his sleep.
- The body temperature drops prior to sleeping, so it is advisable to lower the room temperature (by air conditioners or coolers) so that he can sleep peacefully and more comfortably.
- Restrict the TV watching hours and do not allow him to watch TV for more than 2 hours in a day.
- Do not give him tea or coffee before bedtime. It is advisable to give him milk too one hour before he sleeps.
- Let the child go to the bathroom before he sleeps and put him to sleep in a cosy bed so that he can sleep unrestricted and undisturbed.
- Avoid keeping a TV in the child's bedroom so that he doesn't switch it on when you go out putting him to sleep.
- Avoid taking the child to late night parties or leaving him alone at home on a regular basis. It is advisable to go to such parties for not more then thrice a week. Your good example can create good habits in him and have a positive influence on the child.
- The child should ideally have his dinner at least two hours before he goes to sleep.
- Encourage the child to watch knowledgeable programmes instead of daily soaps on TV so that such programmes (Discovery Channel, History Channel, and National Geographic Channel) contribute towards a healthy mind and he is able to sleep soundly as well.

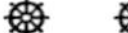

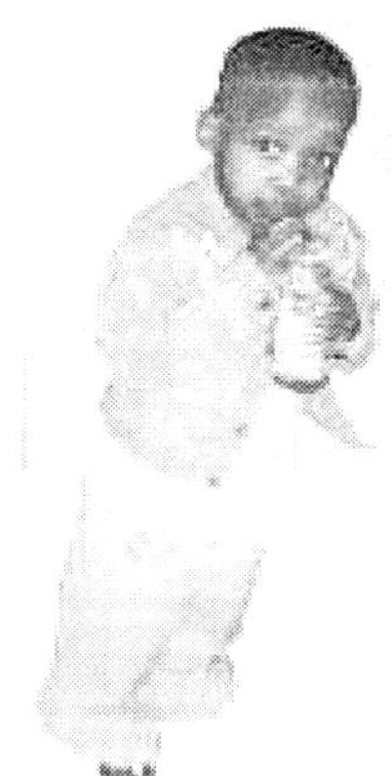

22
LACK OF SELF-CONFIDENCE

Many times, it has been seen that some children lack in self-confidence so much so that when they grow up they are not able to become successful individuals. Children who lack self-confidence also lag behind in their studies.

Child specialist Dr. A. Sethi says, "Self-confidence in children should be developed right from childhood. Only children with self- confidence grow into successful individuals." Mayur is a pampered and extremely mischievous boy. His parents love him a lot. At home, he is into mischief or the other. But if some guests come home or if he has to go to somebody's party, nobody can say that he is the same child as he behaves like a frightened cat. In the same way, when he goes out somewhere he starts stammering in fear. Mayur's problem is that due to lack of self-confidence he is unable to face or talk to anyone except his own family people.

Ill-effects of lack of confidence

If children lack self-confidence, then they develop many types of flaws in their personality:

- Due to lack of self-confidence, children don't do well in

their exams, inspite of knowing everything because of which they get less marks.

- Lack of self-confidence is one of the reasons which make children stammer.
- The child is unable to present himself due to lack of self-confidence, therefore people don't take him or his opinions seriously.
- Lack of self-confidence is also the reason due to which the children develop an inferiority complex.
- A child lacking of self-confidence is unable to face problems or difficult situations and starts panicking.
- If the child doesn't have self-confidence then his growth is not balanced, because of which his health and his mental development are badly affected.
- Lack of self-confidence is also the reason why a child doesn't grow into a successful individual.
- Due to lack of self-confidence some children develop quarrel- some nature and get into fights with their classmates without any reason.
- Children who lack self-confidence even hesitate to go in front of a new person. If they have to talk to a stranger, then they cannot talk properly.
- Lack of confidence can be easily seen in a child's personality. His odd behaviour sometimes makes him a laughing stock.
- Lack of confidence also is the reason for incapability of taking immediate/instant decisions.

REASONS FOR LACK OF SELF-CONFIDENCE

- **Frequent Scolding**

If in a home everybody beats or scolds the child for each and everything, the child starts losing self-confidence. He is not able to understand whether he is doing the right thing or the wrong thing. Each time when he starts to do thing, he starts thinking, whether it is right or wrong and if he will be scolded for it.

- **Neglecting one child**

If at home, one child is loved more, then the other child is neglected and he starts losing his self-confidence. He feels that he is a good for nothing because of which nobody loves him. This is observed in most of the households where the elder child is loved more and the younger one is neglected. This happens more in houses where both the children are either boys or girls.

- **Too much Discrimination between a Boy and a Girl**

In Indian families, it is mostly seen that a boy is given more importance than a girl. All the love and concentration is on the development and education of the boy. Because of this many a times, girls lack self-confidence and also develop inferiority complex. Girls brought up in such an environment not only become victims of inferiority complex in children but also when they grow up and get married; they show the same discrimination towards their children as well. Such girls develop a different type of feeling for boys. Girls brought up in this environment mostly don't become successful as they are unable to attain high qualification and stand on their own feet.

- **Comparison Among Children**

If a child is compared with his own brothers or sisters then also the child may develop lack of self-confidence. Chintu always used to top in his class. His neighbour Jatin was his friend and also his classmate. Jatin was not that good in studies. When both of them would enter the class together, the classteacher would tauntingly say you are always together, come to school together, why can't you study in the same way? At home Jatin's parents would say, "Have you seen? This time also Chintu has stood first in the class, you are good for nothing. Learn something from him. If you cannot come first, then at least try to come with in 4-5 ranks." Jatin started getting irritated. His friendship with Chintu was broken. Gradually he started losing his self-confidence and instead of getting more marks, he started failing in many subjects.

- **Always finding faults with decision of the child**

If a responsibility is given to the child and when he does it in his own way, and then if it is always pointed out that he was wrong, then also the child loses his self-confidence and unable to take a right decision at the right time.

- **Discussing about the behaviour of the child in front of a third person**

When a friend or a relative visits your house and if you tell them about your child's habit to them like he is shy, doesn't talk etc. then the child thinks he is being appreciated and starts behaving in the same way before others. When he goes in front of his strangers he starts biting his nails, lowers, hides himself in a corner or doesn't go and talk to anyone. This behaviour shows his lack of self-confidence.

HOW TO AWAKE SELF-CONFIDENCE IN CHILDREN

Dr. Walia says, "For the proper development in the child, he should be brimming with self-confidence. This makes him successful in his school and later in his life as well. The child should not lack self-confidence and if it has already happened, then these rules/suggestions can be adhered to in order to increase his self-confidence:

- Always appreciate the good and correct work of the child.
- If the child is scolded for a wrong thing then make him understand the difference between right and wrong.
- If you have more than one child, then love all of them equally; never neglect one at the cost of the other.
- Do not compare the child with anyone, even it is with his brother or sister or friend.
- Appreciate the child if he learns something new.
- If you don't have faith in the child's decision making powers, then give him complete instructions and get the things done.
- Try to motivate the child to take his own decisions. If he is in doubt then help him to come to a proper decision after explaining to him the difference between right and wrong.
- Do not discuss about the behaviour of the child in front of others. Praise the child in front of them. This increases the self-confidence and determination of the child.
- Do not discriminate between a boy and a girl. Give them equal love and care so that they turn out into outstanding citizens.

❁ ❁

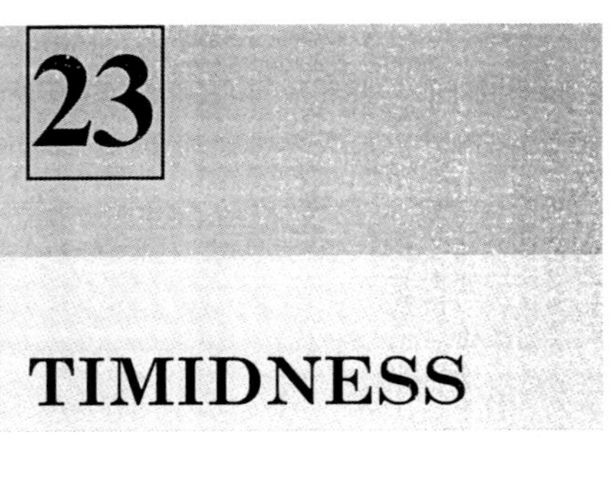

23 TIMIDNESS

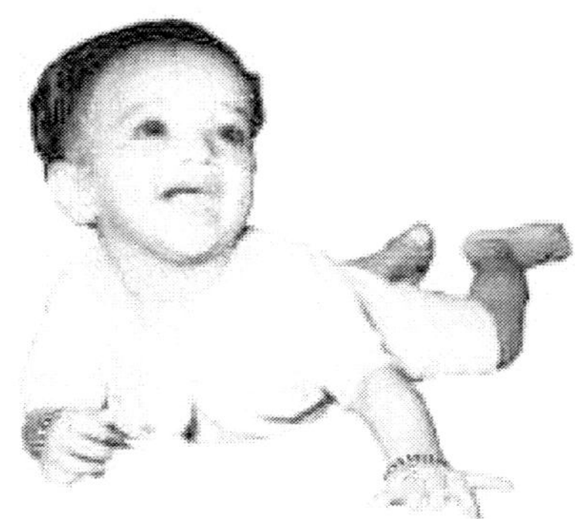

Some children are naturally brave. They are fearless and never hesitate to get involved in bravery acts or even quarrels. Some children on the other hand, are shy and of a quiet temperament, while some are extremely timid by nature.

Types of fear

- Different children have different types of fear.
- Some timid children get extremely frightened whenever they see a horrifying scene in their dream.
- Some children get scared when they witness a violent or unpleasant sequence or a wild, ferocious animal on television.
- Some children get completely engulfed in fear when they happen to witness a mishap or accident so much that at times they lose control over their urinary bladder and pass urine then and there.
- Children who get frightened easily are afraid to sit on a swing, see-saw etc. They never enjoy an adventurous travel or ride because of their inner fear.

- Some children are afraid of stepping into water or swimming while some children exhibit a fear of heights.
- Faint hearted or timid children are afraid of going to the bathroom alone during the night or are afraid of stepping out of their room or house in the night. Such children are in fact scared of darkness.
- Some children are afraid of the sound of crackers, which are burst during Diwali. They are also afraid of bursting crackers themselves.
- Some children are afraid of the bright colours that are used during the festival of Holi. They are so scared that they hide in their rooms during the festival.
- Some children are scared of sleeping alone in their rooms. They refuse to go to their rooms unless they are accompanied by their mother or brother or sister. The mother or the sister has to sit by their side till they go to sleep.

Thus there are different types of fear in children. Some other fears are - the fear of being bitten by a mosquito or ant, the fear of lightning, the fear of getting drenched in the rain and so on.

Mother's Attitude

Generally a newborn gets startled by slightest sound or disturbance around him and starts shaking or moving. But superstitious mothers suspect some external, power or a wicked eye is causing the child to get scared time and again. They start keeping an iron knife under the pillow or bed of the young one as they believe that this would ward of the evil eye. Thus when the child grows up and observes these things, he too starts believing in such things and gets frightened.

In reality however not only do the timid children get frightened and troubled in certain uncommon situations, but they trouble their family members as well.

CAUSES

According to child psychologist Dr. Sushma Bijlani there is always a definite reason behind the feeling of fear in children. Upbringing plays a very important role influencing the actions, behaviour and feelings of the child. Dr. Sushma cited the example of her patients who had come to her for treatment. The patient was a young lady who appeared to be extremely confident in her behaviour and speech. But she mentioned that she was very scared of sleeping alone in her room at night. In the course of the following conversation with Dr. Sushma, she revealed that when she was a kid her mother used to ask her to go to bed quickly and say that an owl will come and bite her if she didn't. At that time she used to quickly cover her face with a blanket or bed sheet and sleep. Even now as she is about to sleep she is reminded of the same fear and she still sleeps covering her face. Dr. Bijlani enumerates the following reasons for fear in children:

- **Witnessing or experiencing an accident during childhood**

If a child happens to witness a mishap in his family or elsewhere during the age of 2-9 years, the terror or fear of the same incident leaves a deep impression on him. The fear surfaces again and again even as he grows up.

Priyansh was a brave child. Once he was travelling in a train with his parents and aunt, when he was five years of age. Suddenly there was a blast in the train. It was a major accident and Priyansh lost his father in the blast. He saw blood and horrifying scenes all around him. He could still hear the cries of the people echoing in his ears even years after the accident. He was so shaken by the incident that he was terrified of sleeping into a bus or a train even as he grew up.

Such incidents shake the confidence of children and make them timid for life.

• Upbringing

As I have also reiterated earlier, upbringing of the child is determining factor in carving out his personality. Upbringing constitutes the values given by the parents as well as by the other close family members such as brother, sister, grandparents, uncle, aunt etc. His behaviour and personality is the sum total of all he sees around him. Apart from this, a healthy environment of the school and the behaviour of the teachers also contribute towards making the child an ideal citizen.

If the child is frightened by the concept of ghosts, wild animals or any such thing to make him do a thing, then the impressionable and innocent mind of the child imbibes the fear forever.

I have seen people avoiding to step out of their house/office in rain and thunder as they fear that lightning might strike at them. Such people can never enjoy a drizzle or a pleasant weather for the fear of lightning. Children of such parents are bound to be timid.

• If either parent is timid or faint-hearted

Generally many women are timid by virtue of their nature. They have no independence in taking their own decisions or to go to college alone etc. When such women become mothers, they instill a similar type of fear in their children as well. They scare the child using the pretext of ghosts and such other things.

In this situation it is but natural for these children to grow up being timid. However, it is not only the women who are faint-hearted. Certain men too might appear to be tough on the outset but are extremely emotional and faint-hearted with respect to their children. If they are scared of swimming or enjoying rides and swing etc. they will try to cultivate a fear for their child as well for the same. Later on the child's fear is attributed to his genes, whereas it has been unnecessarily cultivated externally.

Some mothers are scared of watching action sequences on the television and but naturally they do not let their children watch such movies or scenes. They either switch off the T.V. or cover the eyes of the child when such scenes come on T.V. These things make the child fear normal film scene as well.

- **Lack of natural environment**

If the child happens to be the only child and he has not been provided a natural environment for playing and development, he will end up being a timid and submissive child.

Parents and grandparents tend to worry more for single children. Thus they keep an extremely watchful eye on the child and lay a lot of restrictions and prohibitions for the child. They fear that the child might injure himself or break a bone while jumping, playing etc. This results in the child becoming incapable of taking small decisions even. Thereby he also starts fearing different things.

- **Unnecessary affection and pampering**

Every child is the centre of his parents lives and parents pay utmost attention towards the needs of the child. But some parents tend to over pamper the child and make him timid. This type of a phenomenon is witnessed more in extremely well-to-do families. Such parents do not let the child step out of the house as they feel the outer environment to be unhygienic and unsafe for the child. They think that the child may catch infection or he may injure himself outside.

Such parents keep a strict vigil on the child's every move and keep scaring and sensitizing him unnecessarily. All this makes the child timid.

SOLUTIONS

It has been scientifically acknowledged that it is very difficult to eliminate the fears that the child develops during his initial childhood. Therefore, it is the duty of every parent to ensure that the child has a natural development and that he does not acquire different fears during his childhood. Dr. Ina Gupta suggests the following measures to prevent the child from becoming timid:

- Never terrorise or scare the child. Never blackmail the child into doing a work by using fear tactics such as the fear of ghosts, spirits, animals etc. It is psychologically wrong to scare the child in any manner. This fear becomes an obstacle in the development of the child.
- If parents have their own inherent fear for certain activities, then they should refrain from influencing the child over the same. Children should be allowed to experience things on their own. Children never develop fear of falling down, darkness, swings etc. on their own. It is the elders who inculcate these fears in the child put of their own experience.
- Love and pamper your child but bear it in mind that your over-protectiveness should not take away a normal growing environment from him. Let him play and enjoy life at his age normally.

- If the child happens to be an unfortunate witness to any mishap or accident, it becomes the duty of the parents and the teachers to bring back the child to normalcy. Make the child understand at the appropriate opportunity the cause behind the accident and also that such incidents occur rarely. Gradually remove the fear from the mind of the child.
- If the child has witnessed a theft, robbery or any violent incident (involving bloodshed), it becomes extremely difficult for him to forget the incident immediately. Such incidents keep resurfacing in the mind and haunt the person concerned for long spells of time. Therefore parents and well-wishers of the child will have to make tireless efforts to normalize the child. It can be a time consuming effort. If the child has been affected so badly that the fear has seeped deep into his conscience, then the help of a child specialist or a psychologist should be sought.
- If the child has hurt himself during playing or in the course of an activity, he begins to fear the activity. For example, if the child has fractured his leg while jumping on the table, it is quite possible that he begins to dread every such activity that is associated with jumping. In such a situation the parents should be careful during the healing stage, but also at the same time they should counsel the child on playing a bit carefully. Parents should not use this accident scare on the child from games and play altogether. If they keep reminding the child about this unpleasant incident time and again and start encouraging T.V., computer instead, then the child will end up being dull and inactive.
- The environment around the child should be such that the child doesn't become timid. If his friends or other relatives are building such negative feelings in him, try to bring the child of the fear in a proper way.

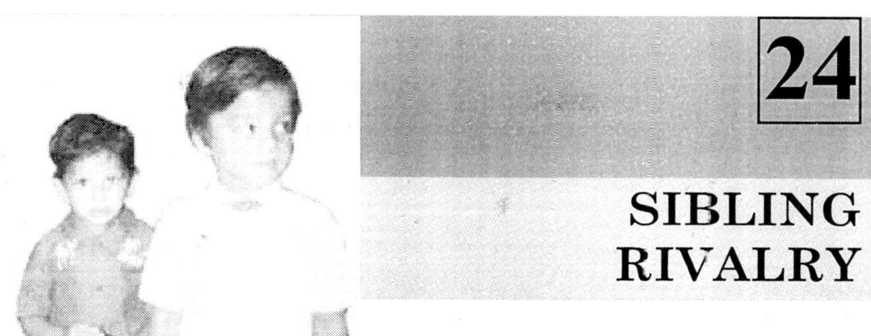

24 SIBLING RIVALRY

It is very common in our families that siblings have conflicts and rivalries. Generally sibling rivalry is more seen in two sisters or two brothers instead of one brother and one sister. If these rivalries are not nipped in the bud, they can aggravate to an irrevocable extent. Good directions from parents make siblings friends but in case of negligence siblings turn into foes.

It is not necessary that siblings, having a little age difference have more conflicts. Sometimes kids even with the age-difference of 6 to 7 years or more have rivalry with their sibling.

Sibling rivalry holds the parents at the centre of the tug. Certainly parents are most responsible in cases of sibling rivalry. They can't escape these conflicts. It is a very usual thing that parents either mother or father favour one or the other child for the little things.

At a very young age, siblings have conflicts over studies, toys, stationery, new clothes, shoes etc. They compare each other for these things. If one of them gets new dress and the other doesn't, he gets jealous and taunts the beneficiary sibling. Then the result is rivalry between them.

Reasons of Rivalry

- If one kid is always compared to his sibling and he is always criticised for his mistakes.
- If one is loved by one and all for the reasons of beauty, intelligence or smartness and the other is neglected or criticised.
- If one sibling is loved more than the other. The reasons may be that he is elder or younger or very weak or has any other problem.
- If one kid is very intelligent and tops his class and the other is poor at studies and first one is always appreciated.
- If one kid gets more rewards from parents, teachers or relatives than the other.
- If elder child doesn't take care for the younger one, then he is rebuked for his carelessness.
- If any partiality is done between siblings.

There may be many such other reasons. They look very trivial issues but it is imperative to solve these fights and conflicts between the siblings right at the beginning. If they are ignored, these may develop into professional rivalry at a later stage. These conflicts hinder the social and personal relationship of the siblings.

Suggestions

The tiny grudges of sibling rivalry look apparently a minor issue. But they may become serious problem. It would be a fault on the part of the parents if they try to sweep the issue under the carpet assuming it to a minor thing. These differences may cause differences between the siblings forever. There are some suggestions-

- Parents should not intervene in the conflicts of kids even if the kids persuade them to do so. Let the kids handle their problem themselves. You should always remember that after a little time, they always patch-up with each other.

- Parents should interfere in the kids' fight only if the situation goes out of control. In the same way, teachers should not intervene in petty fights of their students.
- Parents should deal the siblings' problems and conflicts decisively.
- Parents should always be impartial. They should never take side either of elder or younger or boy. Some parents take side of their daughter taking her to be soft or weak. It is wrong. 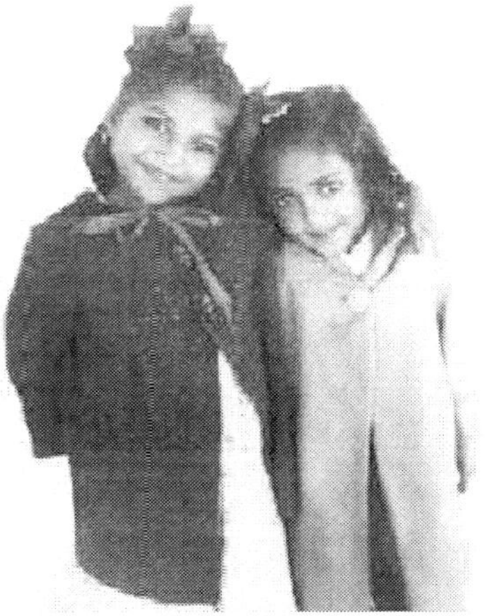
- It is the duty of the parents that they inculcate the feeling of love and regard for their sibling. They should not allow them to fight physically or abuse each other. Children learn these habits from the family atmosphere. So always keep the home atmosphere healthy where everyone has love and regard for other family members. Try to avoid voilence or beating your children and never let the kids do so.
- Parents should not make comparisons between kids.
- Parents should realise that every child has his own qualities and capabilities. So if one child is appreciated for one thing, the other should also be appreciated for his qualities. These comparisons amongst kids breed differences and contempt.
- Parents should create the feeling of responsibility in their kids. Give them responsibilities according to their age. If

elder is given any hard type of work, younger should also be given some work. The feeling of responsibility will make them understand the futility of fights and rivalry.

- Avoid extra attention and favour to any of your kids. This will create the feeling of superior and inferior between them.
- Some families favour their son. Sometimes it may be that he is the only son amongst many sisters. This creates the feeling of envy and jealousy in the hearts of sisters which they might not express in their childhood. But when grown up, it becomes very dangerous for their good relationship. Therefore parents should not favour any child specially. The same thing happens in the families where there is only girl child amongst many brothers. Parents should give equal love and attention to all kids.
- Children should be given freedom to express their feelings to their parents. An open relationship between parents and kids creates healthy atmosphere in the family.
- Parents should encourage their children to work together. Many combined responsibilities can be given to them mutually. For example – they can be directed to clean their room together in one hour. In case of successful completion of responsibility both should be rewarded equally. Thus they will realise the feeling of togetherness and will not have rivalry on trivial things.
- Parents should put a positive outlook in their children. Inculcation of the feeling of love and togetherness will bond them together as good companions. At a tender age, child's mind is easily changed, so try to mould him as a good and loving child.
- All children should be given equal time, love, attention and affection. There should be no bestowal of favours on one child.

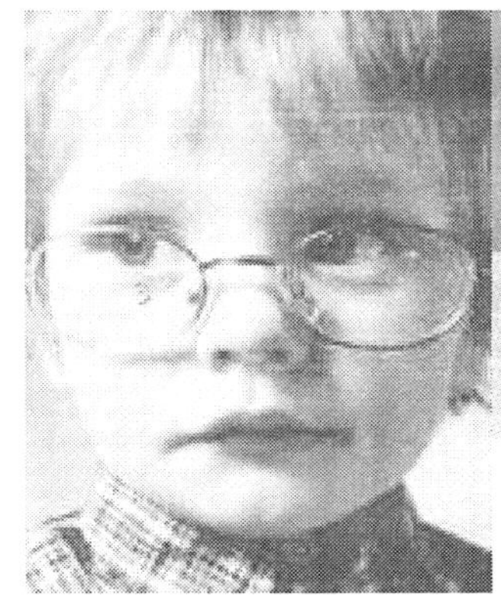

25

OTHER PROBLEMS OF CHILDREN

There can be many other problems with respect to children in addition to those discussed in detail in this book. Some of these can be: crying without any obvious reason, mischievous and adamant child, rebellious and naughty behaviour, the child getting up in the middle of his sleep fairly frightened, vomiting immediately after eating, brightness and intelligence beyond his age, extreme selfishness, cruelty to others etc.

Generally such problems are ignored till such time they do not become pronounced. However, when these problems increase in magnitude and begin to affect the child and others as well, parents naturally become extremely worried and begin to look for solutions.

As we have also discussed earlier, every problem has a definite cause which is rooted either in internal (family etc.) or external circumstances. Therefore it is essential that parents pay attention to the following facts:

- Every child has his own individual personality, liking, disliking, hatred and hobbies. It is not sensible to draw comparisons among different children. No two children have similar physical, mental, behavioural necessities. Also these faculties develop in a varied fashion in different children. Therefore one should never expect a child to behave like any other person or child.

- Children require different kind of assistance at different ages. A two year old would want his mother to pamper and feed him, whereas a five year old wishes to eat his food on a different plate and with his own hands. Therefore, children should be given directions and assistance according to their age and requirement.
- If the child has a problem, then parents should try to find out the causes to the problem so that they can seek a solution to it. After the problem has been sorted out, parents should try to mould the child into a well-behaved and disciplined child.

POSSIBLE CAUSES FOR MANY PROBLEMS OF THE CHILD

There can be many reasons which prompt the child to behave in an unacceptable manner. Some of these reasons can be:

- **Excessive Pampering**

Some parents pamper their children beyond limits and behave as if they are at complete mercy of their children. They fulfil each and every demand of the children irrespective of whether they are reasonable or actually necessary. Naturally children of these kind of parents become shrewd and learn the art of exploiting their parents. They view their parents as a means to fulfil their ends. They never admit their mistakes and view all their demands as reasonable and correct. These children become spoilt brats, adopt bad habits and turn obstinate and naughty.

- **Inability to devote adequate time to children**

The upbringing given by the parents plays a very important role in making the children confident and independent. If parents are always engaged in their work and are unable to devote time to the children and give them proper love and attention, the children are devoid of any feeling of love and affection. These children are mentally unstable and are unable to take decisions at the appropriate time when they grow up. Some fathers feel they fulfil their responsibility if they give money in the house for the child"s necessities. They completely neglect the child and do not give him the love and attention he deserves. But the child perceives the role of the father as someone who talks to him, listens to his tales and stories and plays with him. In the absence of this, the child begins to feel depressed, negative and becomes a victim of many problems at that time.

- **Friction between parents**

Children of parents who constantly keep quarrelling or arguing with each other tend to become naughty and obstinate. In addition to this, if the mother or father is extremely short tempered or loud in their behaviour and create an atmosphere or terror in the house, then it hampers the normal development if the child. The child can become a victim of inferiority complex, rebelliousness or depression or can acquire a destructive or cruel predicament. He can also have a disturbed mindset because of which he can get up in the middle of the sleep frightened and perspiring. The above can begin to hamper his studies and give rise to other problems as well.

- **Not letting the child do his own work**

Some parents do not let their child do any work, even if it is his work and he is capable to doing his own work. They either do his work themselves or deploy servants to do the work. Such parents are of the opinion that they are making the lives of their children simpler and easier. But it has the opposite impact. Such children never get an opportunity of learning about their capabilities. As they never do any work, they never commit mistakes, which are the world's biggest teacher. Such children have no thinking, reasoning or decision making capabilities. In such an environment the children do not get an opportunity to develop qualities of confidence and independence in them. They keep on depending on others for executing their work. This way their urge for self-expression is never fulfilled and they remain dissatisfied in life.

- **Shielding the child at all times**

Some parents have a habit of proving their children right at all occasions and keep praising them endlessly all the time. If the child has fought with someone who comes and complains to the parents about the child, they refuse to accept their child will fight with anyone. Likewise they try to defend their child when he breaks someone's things or brings them home or even eats someone's things. Such a child not only becomes naughty but also learns to tell lies. He comes home and says that he didn't do any mischief and then taking advantage of the situation he starts lying frequently.

- **An unhealthy environment at home**

If in a house there is no mutual love or understanding among parents or frequent and loud disagreements between mother-in-law or other members of the family and each one gives a separate instruction/advice to the child in order to get his or her things done or and to influence the child against the other members. In such a household children learn bad habits very easily. Lying, showing indifferent behaviour towards elders, backbiting, setting up one against the other etc. become very easy for child.

In such households, each person has a separate instruction for the child and it becomes difficult for the child to differentiate between what is wrong and what is right. The child becomes irritable. He becomes uncontrollable, moody and stubborn. Such children sometimes respect their mothers, at other times their fathers and sometimes they have little respect for either of them. A child gets an idea of the outside world only from the atmosphere at his home. In a state of confusion at home he is unable to choose the right path.

Apart from this, there is a yet another aspect of the atmosphere at home which influences the child. If the family members are busy (each in his or her work) and don't care about each other's interest or tastes, don't sit and eat as a family, have no interaction among themselves, the child brought up in such an atmosphere ends up as an extremely selfish and self-absorbed child.

• Neglect of the child

In some households, if there are two children, one child is loved more than the other. The child may be the elder one in some cases and the younger one in some other cases who is shown more love. In such a situation the child who gets less love feels neglected and becomes obstinate, stubborn, irritable and naughty. He also starts faring badly in his studies. He feels that even if he gets good marks he is not appreciated as much as his brother or sister. So he starts losing his self-confidence and develops a feeling of jealousy.

Apart from this, when a new young member (sibling) arrives in the family it often happens that unconsciously everybody's attention shifts on the new one. Whoever comes brings new clothes or toys to the newborn. The elder one in such a case feels extremely neglected. In order to draw everyone's attention on him, he starts biting his nails, sucking his thumb, wets his bed, cries, gets up scared in the middle of night and cries loudly.

• Always pampering the child

In some households, the child is pampered so much that all the members of the family constantly keep an eye on each and every activity of the child. They always try to feed the child something or the other. The child's mother is always coaxing the child to eat one thing or the other. Such a child always makes his parents dance to his tunes. The child understands the weakness of the parents and tries to take advantage of the same and begins to throw tantrums at the very sight of food. He vomits if he is forcibly fed. Due to lack of proper food he becomes weak. He begins to become selective and choosy about food owing to his obstinacy.

- **Indecisiveness of parents**

If the parents are unable to decide what is desirable or not for the child, then proper growth of the child suffers. For example, a child is forbidden to do one thing and the next day nothing is said to him if he does the same thing, dismissing such things as part and parcel of child behaviour. Such type of attitude has a bad influence on the child. He is always in a confused state of mind over whether he will be appreciated or scolded if he does a particular thing. Such a child's mind is always in a state of confusion as to what is wrong and what is right, what should be done, what should not be done etc. The child becomes withdrawn, unresolved and always appears tense. Such a child throws tantrum at any time anywhere, and misbehaves in front of the guests. In the end he has his own way. The child sits down or rolls on the road in front of everyone and ultimately gets what he wants because of his constant crying.

- **Too much strictness or punishments**

It becomes essential to scold the child to teach him discipline. Even otherwise, in order to have a peaceful atmosphere at home, discipline, rules and regulations are very important. But some parents punish the child in order to teach him discipline. If the child slightly disobeys them, he is given strict punishments. This way the child begins to connect discipline only with punishment. Sometimes a child is given very rigid punishments without considering the age of the child, which makes the child extremely obstinate. Discipline taught through cruel punishments or over strictness is useless. This strict discipline makes the child rebellious and headstrong. Besides this, the child starts developing other emotional problems as well.

• A self-centred atmosphere at home

In a house, where each person is a concerned only about himself, that is self centered and is completely unconcerned about what the other person in the family is doing. He ignores other members activities and isn't even aware if they are facing any problems, the child naturally becomes self-centred in such a household. He is in a hurry to fulfil only his interests and wishes without thinking about the problems of others. Such a child becomes totally insensitive towards the trouble he can cause to others in an attempt to satisfy and fulfil his selfish demands. For example, the child will insist on eating an ice-cream or a chocolate in the sweating hot afternoon of the summer months, while the parents are reluctant to go outside because of the weather conditions outside. In a contrasting situation, houses where family members have dinner/lunch together, share jokes, play or indulge in such other group activities, the children too learn the feelings co-operation in a natural way. The children develop a feeling of participating in social life, because of which he participates in the group activities conducted in the school. However, if parents or rather family members keep involved in their own pursuits and pay little or no attention to others, the child too end will up becoming selfish and self-centred.

• Physical disability in the child

If the child keeps falling sick for long intervals or is a victim of physical disability (such as if he is lame, deaf, dwarfish, mute or extremely weak), then he has a number of problems and challenges in to face in his day to day affairs, because of which a many changes occur in his normal behaviour as well. Following problems can surface in his behaviour as a counter reaction to his physical problems – the child might become extremely mischievous, obstinate, rebellious, cruel, harsh, shy, undisciplined and nervous etc.

- **Situations at school**

School plays an extremely important role in influencing the character, behaviour, thoughts and actions of the child. The child comes into the contact of other children and teachers at school. He has an opportunity to learn both good and bad habits from his classmates. The bad habits include telling lies, stealing, fighting, abusing etc.

- **Every child is complete and distinct in his own way**

Most of the times the teachers do not make an attempt to understand child in this perspective. This results in weak children getting neglected as they do not get the attention and sympathy they require and thereby they start losing confidence as well.

- **Teachers do not take an individual interest in the child. They punish the child at slightest mistakes**

In this situation the feelings of inferiority, shame, rebellion and hesitation begin to develop in the child and he becomes adverse towards the idea of going to school to avoid such negative situations altogether.

If the child does not get a healthy mental environment at school and he is subject to insults, inferiority and callousness there, he begins to turn a blind eye towards studies, and behaves rudely with the teachers. Such children begin to misbehave and display undisciplined behaviour. Such children naturally turn into big problems for both parents and teachers. If teachers on their part make an effort to understand the innate natural talents of the child and provide him with an opportunity to harness it, the child will move towards the right direction. In addition to this, the teachers should have an affectionate, sympathetic and loving behaviour with the children keeping in mind the necessities requirements and the individual differences of every child. Children should be given an equal opportunity to express themselves in thoughts and actions according to their age and capability.

- **Parents and other family members prone to telling lies**

If the child has often observed his parents or other family members telling lies, he too will learn the bad habit quite easily. Parents tell their children to make excuses over the phone about the parent not being at home when they are very much there. Lies or excuses such as these, show the path of lies to children.

SOLUTIONS TO THE PROBLEMS

If the parents pay attention to the above reasons which take the child in the wrong direction and make attempts to avoid or eliminate them, then the child can be moulded into an ideal child with a good personality and disciplined behaviour. In brief some solutions are as follows:

1. There is always some reason or the other behind the problems of children. Therefore parents should try and find out the root cause behind the problem.
2. Children too have self-esteem and respect. Therefore respect, appreciate and encourage children as when the situation demands.
3. Pay attention to the child when he is expressing himself and develop independent thinking in him.
4. Express your love to your child every now and then. Also parents and children should have mutual confidence and trust.

5. Peaceful and secure atmosphere is a must for healthy, mental and physical growth of the child.
6. Fulfil the necessities and requirements of the child on time.
7. Praise the child for his individual qualities and talents. Do not compare him with other children.
8. Allot a specific time for games and recreation in the daily routine of the child.
9. Parents should be stable minded. They should always stick to their decisions and be firm when required.
10. Harshness, anger and punishments should not form the basis of discipline. Discipline should be taught on the basis of love and compassion.
11. Physically punishing (beating) the child time and again can turn him into a rebellious and undisciplined child.
12. Medical help should be sought to address the physical problems (or disabilities) of the child and parents should adopt a sympathetic approach towards the child.